"I want to thank the entire NN Live team & faculty for always guiding and helping me throughout my journey. It is a wonderful platform, the best part is that content is regularly updated & prepared by experts. The practice tests are just awesome! Here, learn how to manage time by practicing real time exams. I highly recommend NN Live to all the students who are preparing for nursing competitive exams. Thank you Nursing Next Live for always upgrading our nursing profession" — *Rahul Dahiya* (**Rank-3** *AIIMS NORCET 2020*)

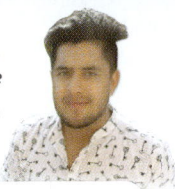

Nursing Next Live
The Next Level of Nursing Education

W0091531

ONE NATION ONE e-RESOURCE

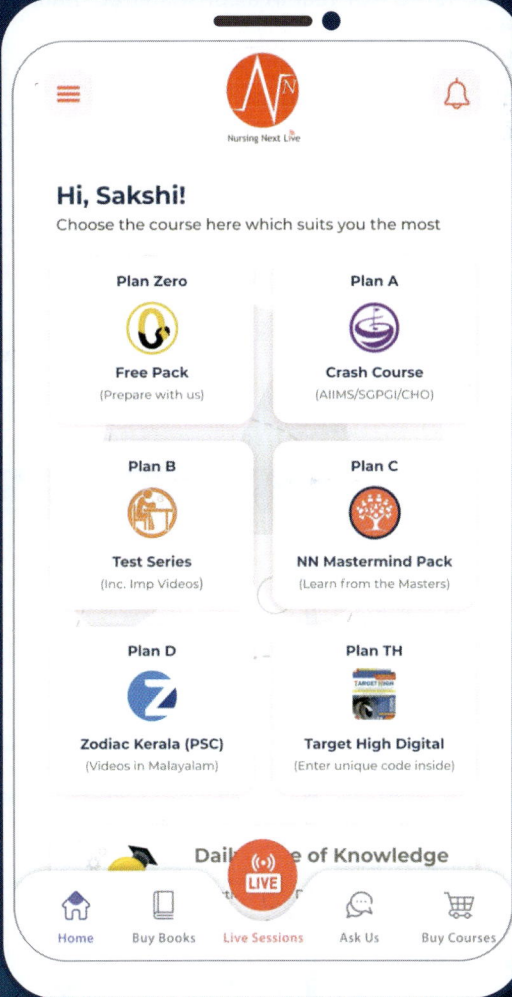

THE COMPLETE PACKAGE

- **40,000+** MCQs with Rationale
- **2000+** Hours of Recorded video lectures (Covering All Subjects/All Topics /Imp Topics Chanting Videos/Exam Discussions/LMR/IBQ & VBQs Discussion)
- **150+** Previous years question papers covering all National & States Level Exams (2020-10)
- Monthly Live Doubt Sessions
- **200+** Newly Created Subject-wise cum Topic-wise Test, Mini Test & Grand Tests based on all important National Exams like AIIMS, PGIMER, JIPMER, DSSSB, RRB & ESIC, also State level exam like Kerala PSC
- **1500+** E-Notes/Flash cards of all the subjects for last minute revision
- **1000+** Image-based Questions with Rationale
- **100+** Video-based Questions with Rationale
- Monthly National Scholarship Test with Rewards points
- **200+** CBS Nursing Books available for purchase
- Scratch & Win Rewards Points and get them redeemed for Buying Books & Nursing Next Packages!

60K USERS | **1000+ CITIES Covered** | **60+ Mins** Average Time users are giving on daily basis | **4.6★ RATINGS** Google Play Store

Unique Features

- Video Download option
- Video & Selective Test Pause & Resume feature
- National Level Ranking
- Review Mode and Practice Mode for attempting test
- Bookmark Your Content for Later Review
- Reattempt of Selective Test Unlimited Times

📞 Helpline and whatsapp number- **9999117411**
(Mon-Sat 9:00 am to 9:00 pm)

✉ Email- **feedback@nursingnextlive.in**

🌐 Web- **www.nursingnextlive.com**

Join Telegram Channel: **NN Live Spreading Knowledge**

New Name, New Interface & in New Platforms
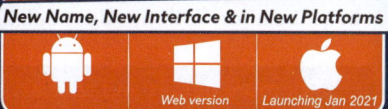
Web version | Launching Jan 2021

Nursing Next Live Pack/Courses

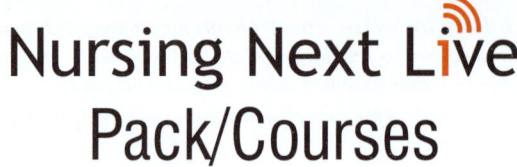

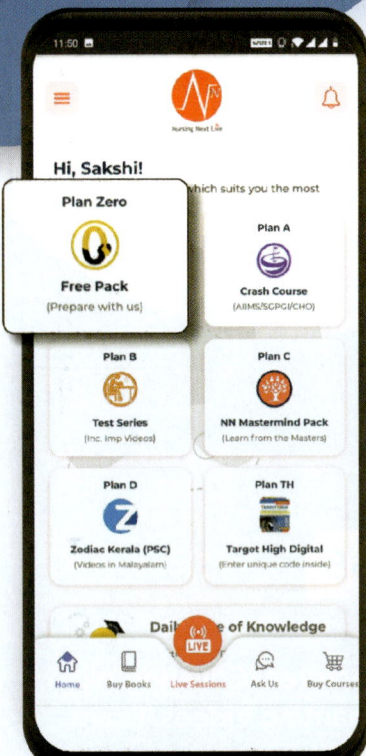

Plan ZERO : FREE Pack (Validity Unlimited)
What all you will get

- **2000+** MCQs with Rationale covering All Subjects, Important Topics
- **150+** E-Notes covering All Subjects, Selective important Topics
- **100+** Hours of Lectures covering All Subjects (Topic-wise/Imp Topics/Chanting/Exam Discussions)
- **100+** IBQS & VBQs of All Subjects
- **15** Most Recent/Previous Year Papers with Rationale (In Attempt/PDF)
- **5+** Grand Test & Bonus Test based on Real Time Exam Pattern
- Daily Dose of Word of the Day, Fact of the Day, Practice Pearls, Question of the Day
- Unsolved & Solved Question Papers of BSc 1st to 4th Year in a consolidated manner covering all Important Universities (Forthcoming)
- Monthly Scholarship Test with Special Prizes & Cash Back
- How to Prepare for Exams in the form of Study Planner/Videos
- Complete Access to Target High Extra Edge Section – which includes additional MCQs & Golden Points in Video Form

For more details and special offers log on to www.nursingnextlive.com

Plan A : Crash Courses (Exam Centric)
What all you will get

Plan A1 – CHO Crash Course (Validity 60 Days)
- **32+** Subject-wise Tests & Grand Tests (including Bonus Tests & Previous Years Papers)
- **1500+** Questions with rationale
- **70+** E-notes for last minutes revision covering all the important topics as per the syllabus of CHO
- **30+** (Duration of 32+ Hours) Pre-recorded Videos given by top faculties in Hinglish covering every important topic from exam point of view

Plan A2 – AIIMS NORCET 2020 Crash Course (Validity 90 Days)
- **60+** Live Tests Subject-wise based on AIIMS Delhi pattern
- **1500+** Qs with Rationale including MCQs, IBQs, VBQs, Clinical skills, Priority setting, and case study
- **15+** Mock Test, Revision Test, and Grand Tests based on Real time pattern of AIIMS Delhi with Negative Marking and National Level Ranking
- All Subject-wise Tests & Grand Tests are with Detailed Rationales
- **140+** Last Minute Revision Notes based on Frequently asked Topics in previous Years
- **12+** Videos on Chanting Session by Top Educators/Subject Experts
- **35+** Multiple videos on special tricks for non-nursing subjects, tips on memory retention, strategies to attempt exams, etc.
- Success Guaranteed as we have had 150+ Selections (Rank 12 to 5k) in AIIMS NORCET 2020.

Plan A3 – Target Kerala PSC Crash Course (Validity 90 Days)
- **60+** Subject-wise/Grand Test with Rationale
- **320+** E-Notes in form of Subject-wise synopsis
- **50+** Hours of Videos in English (Important Topics Pre-loaded video + Chanting videos)
- In association with our Best-Selling Title - Target High Staff Nurse Entrance Exam

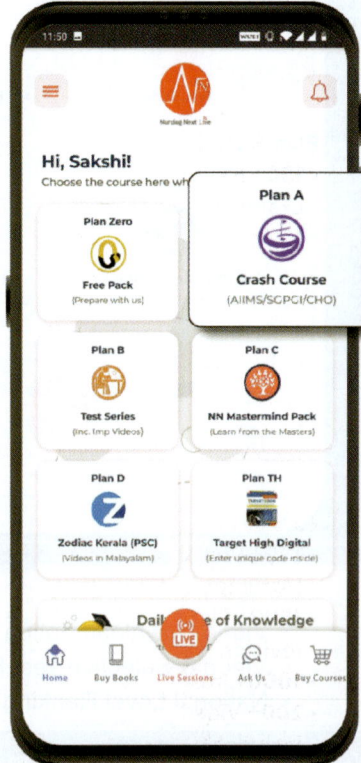

For more details and special offers log on to www.nursingnextlive.com

Plan B:
Test Series Ver 2.0
What all you will get

Plan B 1 Test Series (Duration 6 Months)
- **90+** Newly Created Subject-wise, Mini Test & Grand Test focusing all important National Exams AIIMS, PGIMER, JIPMER, DSSSB, RRB & ESIC (In 6 months)
- **6500+** Qs (MCQs, IBQs, VBQs) with Rationale & updated reference from standard textbooks. All the Tests are designed by the Subject Experts & Topper Students (In 6 months)
- **200+** Hours Recorded Video Lectures of Nursing/Non-Nursing Subjects by some of India's best nursing faculties/subject experts. Lectures are in English/Hindi language focusing on concept-based learning
- **5** Exam Discussion Videos of 2019 Exam papers (Duration 20 Hours)
- **150+** Hours of Recorded Video on Subject-wise Exam Discussion of previous years papers (2017-18) of all nursing exams delivered by subject experts
- **5** Skill Procedure videos demonstrating Nursing Skills in real-time
- **100+** Previous Year Exam Papers of all Nursing Exams from 2020-10 with Rationale (Attempt/View PDF Mode)
- **1500+** Flash cards on all the important topics of all the subjects for last minute revision (In 6 months)
- **800+** Image-based Questions with Rationale
- **150+** Video-based Qs with Rationale
- Includes complete content of current and upcoming crash courses

Plan B 2 Test Series (Duration 12 Months)
- **150+** Newly Created Subject-wise, Mini Test & Grand Test focusing all important National Exams AIIMS, PGIMER, JIPMER, DSSSB, RRB & ESIC (In 12 months)
- **10,000+** Qs (MCQs, IBQs, VBQs) with Rationale & updated reference from standard textbooks. All the Tests are designed by the Subject Experts & Topper Students (In 12 months)
- **200+** Hours Recorded Video Lectures of Nursing/Non-Nursing Subjects by some of India's best nursing faculties/subject experts. Lectures are in English/Hindi language focusing on concept-based learning
- **6** Exam Discussion Videos of 2020 Exam papers (Duration 25 Hours)
- **150+** Hours of Recorded Video on Subject-wise Exam Discussion of previous years papers (2017-18) of all nursing exams delivered by subject experts
- **5** Skill Procedure videos demonstrating Nursing Skills in real-time
- **120+** Previous Year Exam Papers of all Nursing Exams from 2020-10 with Rationale (Attempt/View PDF Mode) (In 12 Months)
- **1500+** Flash cards on all the important topics of all the subjects for last minute revision (In 12 Months)
- **1000+** Image-based Questions with Rationale
- **200+** Video-based Qs with Rationale
  Includes complete content of current and upcoming crash courses

For more details and special offers log on to www.nursingnextlive.com

Nursing Next Live Pack/Courses

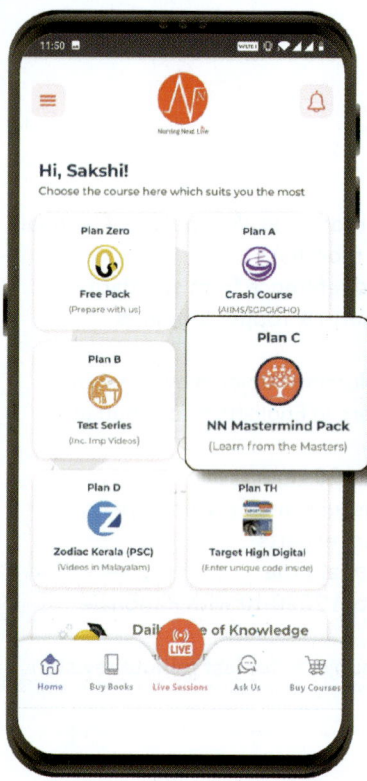

Plan C plus:
Nursing Next MASTERMIND Pack
(One in All, All in One)
Combined Pack - Includes Plan A & B (Validity 12 Months)

Special Features

- Nursing Next's **"NN Mastermind Pack"**, is a **One-Stop solution** for all your exam preparation needs for Staff Nurse Entrance Exams & Nursing Undergraduate Exams!
- It is our **One-in-All, All-in-One** pack for the nursing students of the Digital era!
- NN Mastermind Pack is exactly that 'learning tool' for all the nursing aspirants. It is carefully planned, and strategically designed, under the expertise of TOP Medical/Nursing Educators, just to make learning more authentic and easier for our students.
- Covering All Subjects, All Topics concepts from **Basics to Advance level** pattern with the help of Videos/Question Bank & Handwritten Notes
- The Masterminds (TOP EDUCATORS) of NN Live have focused on **ALL** the upcoming **Nursing Exams** by giving two convenient options of 'Individual pack', or 'Combined (NN Mastermind Pack)'
- **NN Mastermind** Pack is a "road to success" for those who are preparing either for the any and all **staff nurse entrance exams**.

What all you will get

Plan C plus (Inc. Plan A + Plan B)
- **1200+** hours of Video Lectures on All Subject/All Topics
- **11,000+** Questions with Rationale covering All Subject/All Topics
- **IBQs/VBQs** Video Discussions of All Subjects
- Monthly **Live Doubt** Sessions
- Rapid Revision Videos for **AIIMS NORCET 2021** (In July/August'21)
- **Handwritten Notes** of videos in PDF form will be integrated in the app by Feb '21
- Focusing on Quality study over quantity study, using the smart-study approach
- All the Content will be Live in **Four Phases in 4 Months** (Nov-Feb '21)
- All upcoming exams Important Topics & Exam/Discussions will be covered
- Complete 360 Approach for preparation
- Unlimited Time of Watch Time, FREE Download Video option, National Level Ranks, Bookmark the content, Pause & Resume
- **Best Guidance & Support at every stage**
- **+ Plan A of NN Live** (Complete access to Current & Upcoming Crash Courses)
- **+ Plan B of NN Live** (Complete access to Test Series Version 2.0)

Refer to Plan A & B for more details on the content included with Plan C plus

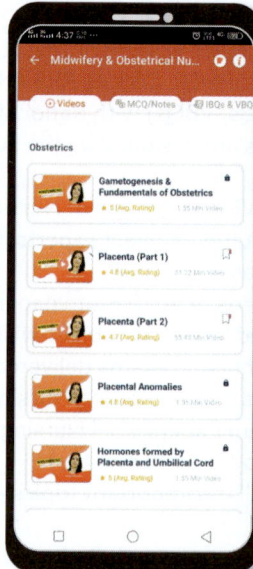
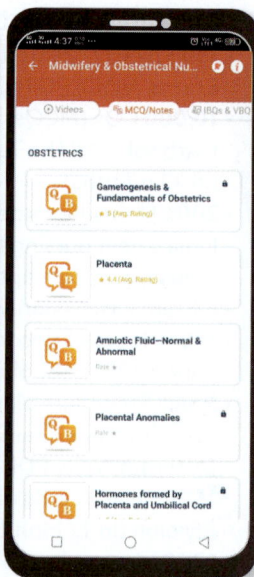

For more details and special offers log on to www.nursingnextlive.com

Nursing Next Mastermind Faculties

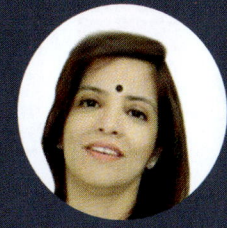
Dr. Sakshi Arora Hans
(Midwifery & Obstetrical Nursing)

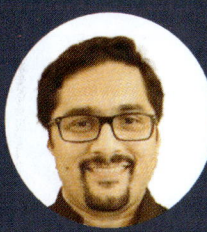
Dr. Rohan Khandelwal
(MSN-Surgery)

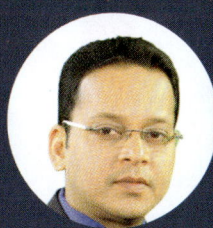
Dr. Ranjan Patel
(Pharmacology)

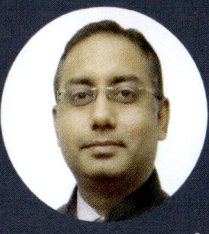
Dr. Mukhmohit Singh
(Community Health Nursing)

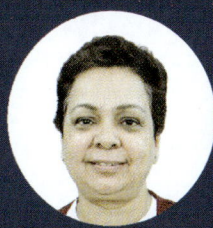
Dr. Shivika Sethi
(Microbiology)

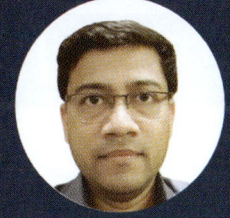
Dr. Ashish Kumar
(Physiology)

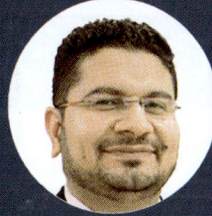
Dr. Aman Setiya
(MSN-Medicine)

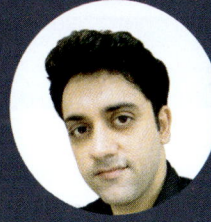
Dr. Anand Bhatia
(Pediatric Nursing)

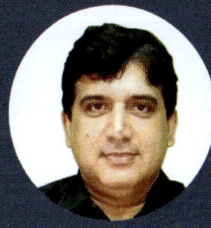
Dr. Dharmendra Singh
(Mental Health Nursing)

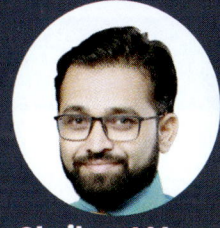
Dr. Shrikant Verma
(Anatomy)

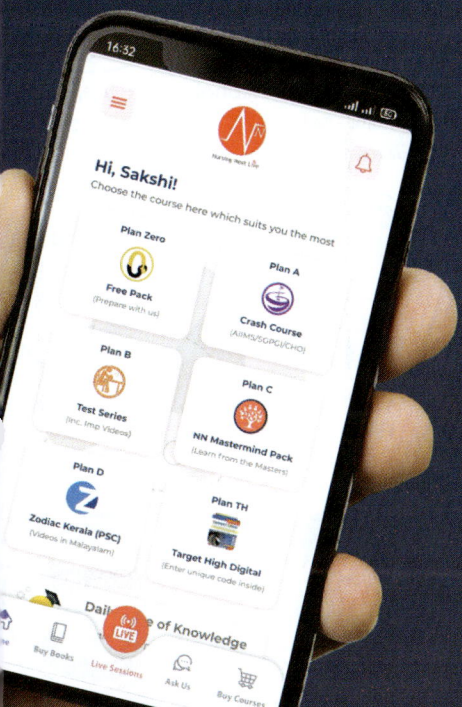

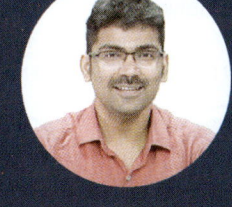
Dr. Karthikeyen Pethusamy
(Biochemistry & Nutrition)

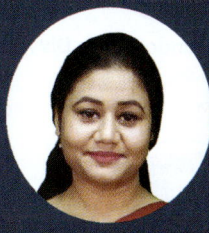
Ms. Sabina Ali
(FON, Nursing Research & Statistics)

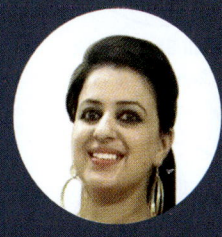
Dr. Mrinalini Bakshi
(General English)

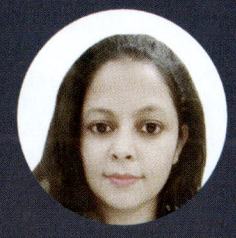
Ms. Priyanka Randhir
(Sociology & Computer)

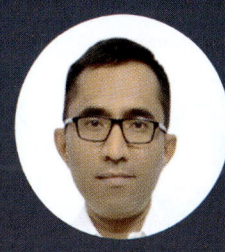
Mr. Nitish Dubey
(General Arithmetic)

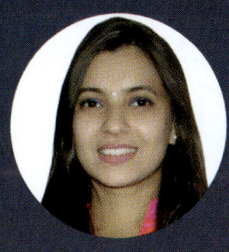
Ms. Saloni Sharma
(Aptitude & Reasoning)

TOP RANK HOLDERS

With over 150+ AIIMS NORCET 2020 Selections &

Say Hello to the
You can

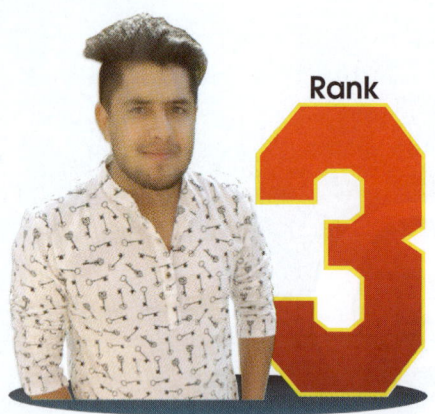
Rank 3
Rahul Dahiya
Roll No. 9016060

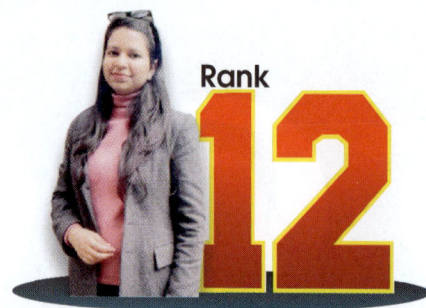
Rank 12
Nisha Singla
Roll No. 9101820

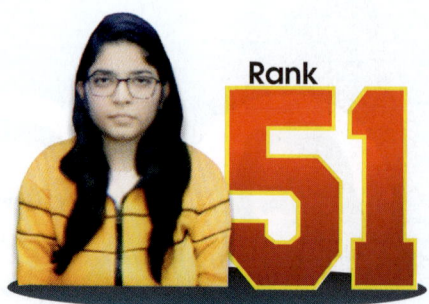
Rank 51
Komal Dhull
Roll No. 9024458

OUR ALL INDIA

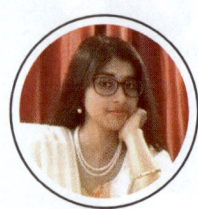
Saswati Bhommick
Rank - 141
Roll No. 9012620

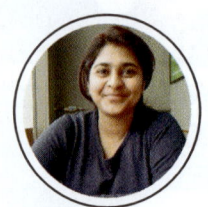
Sohini Mandal
Rank - 145
Roll No. 9042723

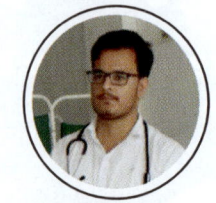
Divyanshu Khandelwal
Rank - 152
Roll No. 9011121

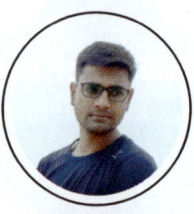
Prithvi Raj
Rank - 171
Roll No. 9030852

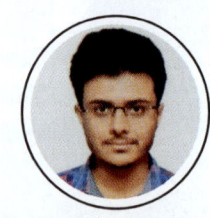
Ch. Prakash Kumar Nanjibhai
Rank - 244
Roll No. 9057267

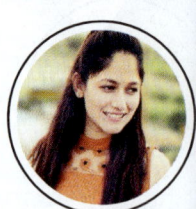
Arti
Rank - 245
Roll No. 9090452

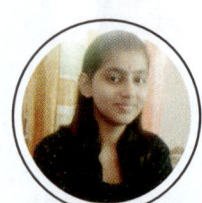
Annu Dahiya
Rank - 390
Roll No. 9005214

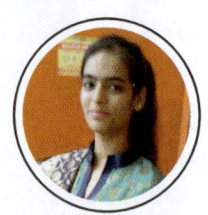
Shipra Choudhary
Rank - 417
Roll No. 9049237

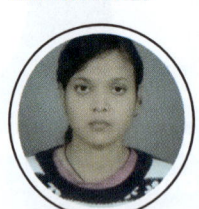
Pragya Maurya
Rank - 466
Roll No. 9033415

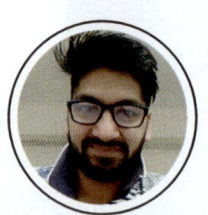
Mohan
Rank - 498
Roll No. 9090721

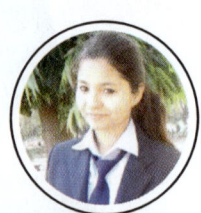
Rinki Negi
Rank - 519
Roll No. 9004223

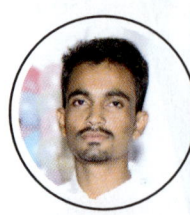
Om Leelawat
Rank - 523
Roll No. 9025575

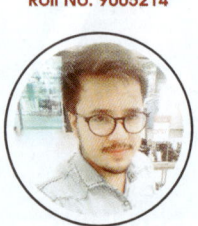
Mohammed Nadim
Rank - 803
Roll No. 9103198

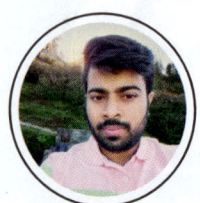
Abhas Singh
Rank - 822
Roll No. 9077010

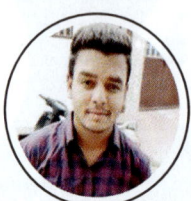
Kartavya Thaker
Rank - 827
Roll No. 9054007

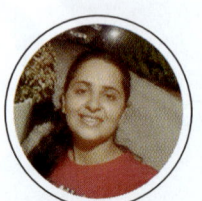
Sunita Goswami
Rank - 843
Roll No. 9060327

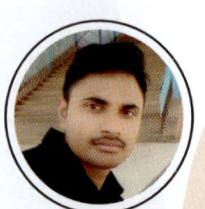
Dinesh Gehlot
Rank - 923
Roll No. 9043284

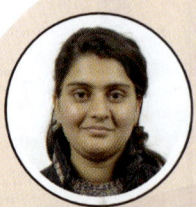
Surabhi Nandwana
Rank - 939
Roll No. 9091040

# of Nursing Next Live

1000+ students who cleared the nursing exams

NursingNextSquad!
be the Next . . .

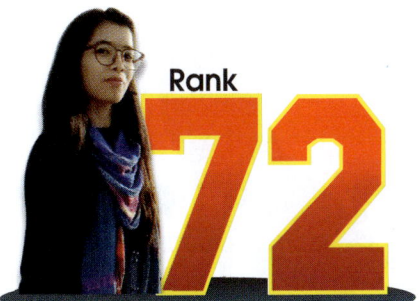
Rank 72
Shivani Bourai
Roll No. 9092877

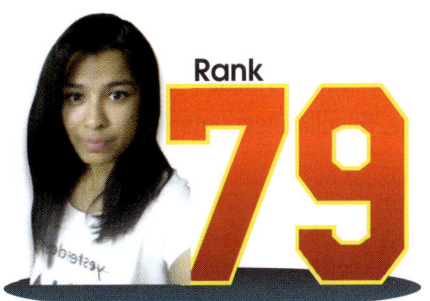
Rank 79
Nivedita Saini
Roll No. 9004587

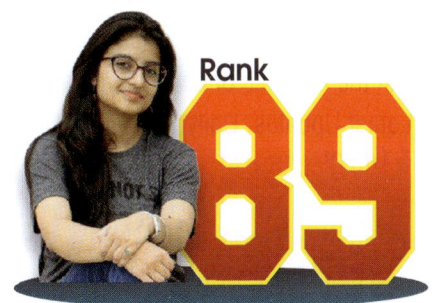
Rank 89
Rupali Garg
Roll No. 9054544

TOP RANKERS

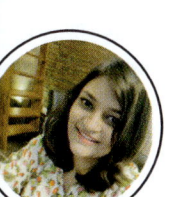
Mamta
Rank - 297
Roll No. 9063879

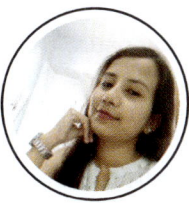
Neelam Rana
Rank - 326
Roll No. 9089800

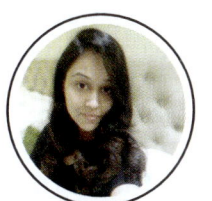
Gargi Baruah
Rank - 336
Roll No. 9019608

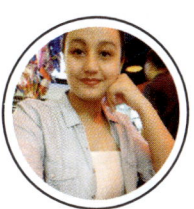
Parul Vats
Rank - 338
Roll No. 9027211

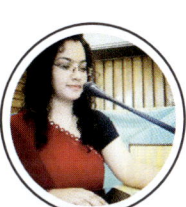
Anjali Chauhan
Rank - 367
Roll No. 9053536

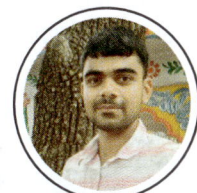
Vishal Gupta
Rank - 384
Roll No. 9023854

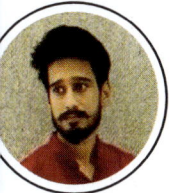
Sri Bhagwan
Rank - 540
Roll No. 9054478

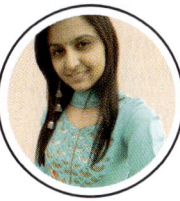
Jyoti Dhull
Rank - 560
Roll No. 9052005

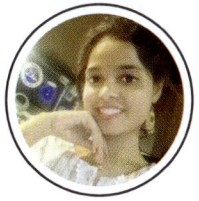
Sonia Mandal
Rank - 584
Roll No. 9007042

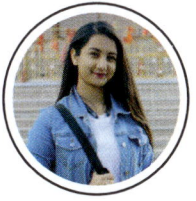
Pratibha Jhagta
Rank - 585
Roll No. 9093660

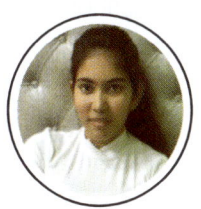
Arpita Pandey
Rank - 624
Roll No. 9087198

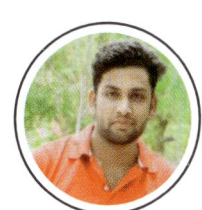
Vikram Prakash Kumhar
Rank - 745
Roll No. 9045800

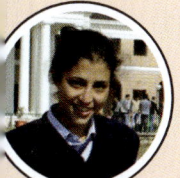
Ritu Tiwari
Rank - 947
Roll No. 9066617

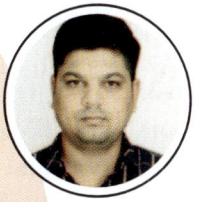
Himalay Choudhary
Rank - 1063
Roll No. 9094287

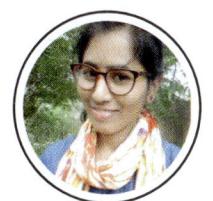
Swapnal Mallinath Sarne
Rank - 1197
Roll No. 9031619

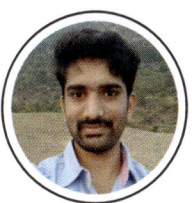
D.V. Ganapthi
Rank - 1317
Roll No. 9017393

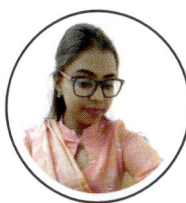
Varsha
Rank - 1330
Roll No. 9092296

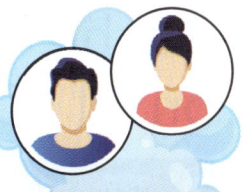
You Will Be The Next...

Why Follow Nursing Next Live On Social Media

Join our Telegram Channel

- Telegram Channel name: **NN Live Spreading Knowledge**
- EXCLUSIVE Content for both PAID and FREE Subscribers
- Get the Glimpse of all the Content MCQS, IBQs, E-Notes, Videos
- Latest Updates, Daily Dosage of Learning, Quiz, Special Discounts & Offers

Subscribe to our YouTube Channel

- YouTube Channel name: **Nursing Next Live**
- Watch Videos on 'Success Stories & get some special Preparation Tips and Tricks' from our Top Rank Holders of AIIMS NORCET 2020
- Watch Latest Videos of all Subjects/Importand Topics by Top Educators & mastermind faculties
- Various Last Minute Revision, Chanting videos before the exams
- Watch Motivational Videos & Live Doubt Sessions every month for Paid Subscribers

Like us and Follow our Facebook page

- Facebook Page name: **Nursing Next Live**
- Get Latest Updates & Discount Offers
- Read Students Feedbacks & Testimonials
- Fun & Learn Activities - Participate and win exciting prizes & free subscriptions

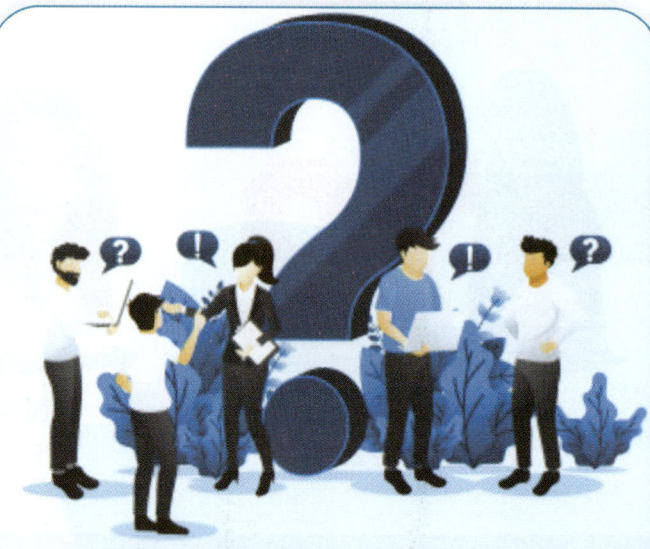

24×7 Guidance & Support

We provide personalized guidance and counseling to all our Subscribers, to ensure that their preparation is in the right direction, that is, toward success. That's why we have an active support service, handled especially by our:

- **Nursing Counselors/Academic Counselors –** To suggest you what to refer as per your need and want
- **Relationship Managers –** To guide you throughout your learning journey and help you at each step
- **Guidance & Counselor -** To teach you what to study and how to study
- **Scientific Team –** To clear your Scientific Doubts within **24-48 Hours**

Nursing Next Live
will be available for use on all of your devices

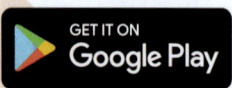 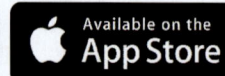

Coming Soon

How to connect with us?

- Any Doubt, Ask Us – (In App Support 24x7)
- Helpline and WhatsApp no: **9999117411** (Mon-Sat 9:00 am to 8:00 pm, Sunday 9:00 am to 2:00 pm)
- Email: **feedback@nursingnextlive.in**
- Web: **www.nursingnextlive.com**

Practical Record Book of
Psychiatric Nursing

For BSc and Post Basic BSc Nursing Students

As per the Syllabus of Indian Nursing Council

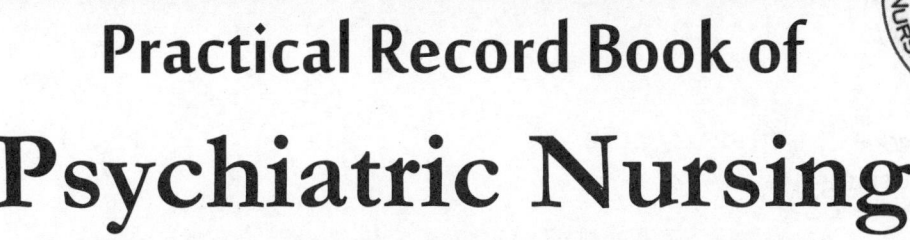

Prof. Ramandeep Kaur Dhillon MSc, PhD(MHN)
Principal
Ajit Nursing Institute
Sunam, Punjab

Deepak Shandilya RN RM, MSc (MHN), PhD
Professor cum Vice- Principal
Desh Bhagat University College of Nursing
Punjab

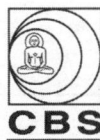

CBS Publishers & Distributors Pvt Ltd

• New Delhi • Bengaluru • Chennai • Kochi • Mumbai • Kolkata
• Hyderabad • Pune • Nagpur • Patna • Vijayawada

Practical Record Book of
Psychiatric Nursing
For BSc and Post Basic BSc Nursing Students

ISBN: 978-93-88108-80-5

Copyright © Authors & Publishers

First Edition: 2019

All rights reserved. No part of this book may be reproduced or transmitted in any form or by any means, electronic or mechanical, including photocopying, recording, or any information storage and retrieval system without permission, in writing, from the authors and the publishers.

Published by **Satish Kumar Jain** and produced by **Varun Jain** for

CBS Publishers and Distributors Pvt Ltd
4819/XI Prahlad Street, 24 Ansari Road, Daryaganj, New Delhi 110 002, India.
Ph: 23289259, 23266861, 23266867   Website: www.cbspd.com
Fax: 011-23243014
e-mail: delhi@cbspd.com; cbspubs@airtelmail.in.

Corporate Office: 204 FIE, Industrial Area, Patparganj, Delhi 110 092
Ph: 4934 4934   Fax: 4934 4935
e-mail: bhupesharora@cbspd.com

Branches

- **Bengaluru:** Seema House 2975, 17th Cross, K.R. Road,
  Banasankari 2nd Stage, Bengaluru 560 070, Karnataka
  Ph: +91-80-26771678/79   Fax: +91-80-26771680
  e-mail: bangalore@cbspd.com

- **Chennai:** No. 7, Subbaraya Street, Shenoy Nagar, Chennai 600 030, Tamil Nadu
  Ph: +91-44-42032115   Fax: +91-44-42032115
  e-mail: chennai@cbspd.com

- **Kochi:** Ashana House, 39/1904, AM Thomas Road, Valanjambalam, Eranakulam 682 018, Kochi, Kerala
  Ph: +91-484-4059061-62-64-65   Fax: +91-484-4059065
  e-mail: kochi@cbspd.com

- **Kolkata:** No. 6/B, Ground Floor, Rameswar Shaw Road, Kolkata-700014 (West Bengal), India
  Ph: +91-33-2289-1126, 2289-1127
  e-mail: kolkata@cbspd.com

- **Mumbai:** 83-C, Dr E Moses Road, Worli, Mumbai-400018, Maharashtra
  Ph: +91-22-24902340/41   Fax: +91-22-24902342
  e-mail: mumbai@cbspd.com

Representatives

- Hyderabad   +91-9885175004
- Patna   +91-9334159340
- Mangalore   +91-9741432102
- Nagpur   +91-8424005858
- Vijayawada   +91-74069-04007

Printed At : Goyal Offset Printers

Dedicated to

Almighty God
Our loving parents, families, teachers, students, friends
and nursing professionals

Preface

Psychiatric Nursing/Mental Health Nursing is concerned with the care of infants, children, adults and geriatric population. It focuses on providing comprehensive care to all segments of life. The goal of mental health is to promote optimum state of physical, mental and social wellbeing.

This record book contains information specifically designed to assist nursing students in clinical practice. Its primary purpose is to assist nursing students in clinical assignments.

The Practical Record Book of Psychiatric Nursing for BSc and Post Basic BSc Nursing Students provides quality content regarding Mental Health Nursing practicals and it follows the syllabus as per the Indian Nursing Council (INC).

Nowadays, students of nursing are trapped in very busy academic schedule. This record book will help the students in completing clinical assignments, and will guide and instruct the students step-by-step for completing their assignments. It will also reduce the workload of clinical instructors and teachers while guiding the students during their practical assignments.

Each task (assignment) is dealt with the example followed by format for accomplishing assignments.

This book is useful for the Mental Health BSc/Post Basic BSc Nursing students.

We hope that this record book will be liked by nursing students and faculties. We also earnestly invite suggestions and comments of the readers about the book.

Prof. Ramandeep Kaur Dhillon
Deepak Shandilya

Acknowledgments

Deep sense of gratitude to Almighty God for providing us with abundant blessings and strength, and helping us in all accomplishments.

Our sincere thanks to all our teachers who have guided and polished our ideas in the touchstone of their experience and knowledge.

We are very thankful to all our colleagues and friends for their constant support.

We extend our thanks to our parents for shaping our career in nursing profession. Without their blessings and guidance, it was an uphill task to accomplish it successfully.

We convey our sincere thanks to **Mr Satish Kumar Jain** (Chairman) and **Mr Varun Jain** (Managing Director), M/s CBS Publishers and Distributors Pvt Ltd for their wholehearted support in publication of this record book. We have no words to describe the role, efforts, inputs and initiatives undertaken by **Mr Bhupesh Arora**, Vice-President, (Publishing and Marketing), PGMEE and Nursing Division for helping and motivating us.

We would like to thank Dr Mrinalini Bakshi (Sr Content Developer and Editor) for her editorial support on this project. We personally thank Ms Nitasha Arora (Project Manager), Mr Nitish K Dubey (Senior Editor) and all the production team members Mr Ashutosh Pathak, Mr Phool Kumar, Mr Bunty Kashyap, Mr Prakash Gaur, Mr Chaman Lal, Ms Tahira Parveen, Ms Babita Verma, Mr Chander, Mr Raju Sharma, Mr Manoj Chaudhary, Mr Vikram Chaudhary, Mr Manoj Malakar and Ms Manorma for devoting laborious hours in designing and typesetting of the record book.

Syllabus

MENTAL HEALTH NURSING/ PSYCHIATRIC NURSING
BSc NURSING
PRACTICAL

Placement: Third Year
Fourth Year

Time: Practical: 270 hours (9 weeks)
Internship — 95 hours (2 weeks)

Areas	Duration (in week)	Objectives	Skills	Assignments	Assessment method
Psychiatric OPD	1	□ Assess patients with mental health problems □ Observe and assist in therapies □ Counsel and educate patient, and families	□ Health taking □ Perform mental status examination (MSE) □ Assist in Psychometric assessment □ Perform Neurological examination □ Observe and assist in therapies □ Teach patients and family members	□ History taking and Mental status examination-2 □ Health education-1 □ Observation report of OPD	□ Assess performance with rating scale □ Assess each skill with checklist □ Evaluation of health education □ Assessment of observation report □ Completion of activity record.
Child Guidance clinic	1	□ Assessment of children with various mental health problems □ Counsel and educate children, families and significant others	□ History taking □ Assist in psychometric assessment □ Observe and assist in various therapies □ Teach family and significant others	□ Case work-1 □ Observation report of different therapies-1	□ Assess performance with rating scale □ Assess each skill with checklist □ Evaluation of the observation report
Impatient ward	6	□ Assess patients with mental health problems □ To provide nursing care for patients with various mental health problems □ Assist in various therapies	□ History taking □ Perform mental status examination (MSE) □ Perform Neurological examination □ Assist in psychometric assessment	□ Give care to 2–3 patients with various mental disorders □ Case study-1 □ Care plan-2 □ Clinical presentation 1	□ Assess performance with rating scale □ Assess each skill with checklist

Contd...

Areas	Duration (in week)	Objectives	Skills	Assignments	Assessment method
		<ul><li>Counsel and educate patients, families and significant others</li></ul>	<ul><li>Record therapeutic communication</li><li>Administer mediations</li><li>Assist in Electro-convulsive Therapy (ECT)</li><li>Participate in all therapies</li><li>Prepare patients for Activities of Daily living (ADL)</li><li>Conduct admission and discharge counselling</li><li>Counsel and teach patients and families</li></ul>	<ul><li>Process recording 2</li><li>Maintain drug book</li></ul>	<ul><li>Evaluation of the case study, care plan, clinical presentation, process recording</li></ul>
Community psychiatry	1	<ul><li>To identify patients with various mental disorders</li><li>To motivate patients for early treatment and follow up</li><li>To assist in follow up clinic</li><li>Counsel and educate patient, family and community</li></ul>	<ul><li>Conduct case work</li><li>Identify individuals with mental health problems</li><li>Assists in mental health camps and clinics</li><li>Counsel and Teach family members, patients and community</li></ul>	<ul><li>Case work-1</li><li>Observations report on field visits</li></ul>	<ul><li>Assess performance with rating scale</li><li>Evaluation of case work and observation report</li><li>Completion of activity record</li></ul>

POST BASIC BSc NURSING
PRACTICAL

The student will be provided opportunity to
- Observe record and report the behavior of their selected patients.
- Record the process of interaction.
- Assess the nursing needs of their selected patients. Plan and implement the nursing intervention.
- Counsel the attendant and family members of patient.
- Participate in the activities of psychiatric team.
- Write observation report after a field visit to the following places:
  - Child guidance clinic.
  - School/Special Schools (For mentally subnormal]. Mental Hospital.
  - Community mental health centres
  - De-addiction centre.

Contents

Contents	Page Nos
TERMINOLOGIES	1
PROCEDURES	10
Admission and Discharge	
Format 1	12
Format 2	15
Format 3	18
Orthostatic Hypotension	21
Format 1	23
Format 2	27
Format 3	31
Oral Medication	35
Format 1	38
Format 2	42
Format 3	46
Electroconvulsive Therapy (ECT)	50
Format 1	54
Format 2	59
Format 3	64
Restraining	69
Format 1	73
Format 2	76
Format 3	79
Example of History Taking	85
Format of History Taking/Collection	91-120
Format 1	91
Format 2	99
Format 3	106

Contents	Page Nos
Format 4	113
Format 5	120
Example of Mental Status Examination	127-164
Format 1	136
Format 2	150
Format 3	164
Example of Mini Mental Status Examination	178
Format of Mini Mental Status Examination	179-183
Format 1	179
Format 2	181
Format 3	183
Example for Process Recording	185
Format of Process Recording	189-197
Format 1	189
Format 2	193
Format 3	197
Example of Nursing Care Plan	201
Format of Nursing Care Plan	212-258
Format 1	212
Format 2	235
Format 3	258
Example of Case Study	281
Format of Case Study	289-304
Format 1	289
Format 2	304
Example of Case Presentation	319
Format of Case Presentation	320

STUDENT'S PROFILE

Paste your
Passport size Photo

Name of the Student : _____

Reg. No./Enroll No. : _____

Course/Year : _____

Subject : _____

Batch : _____

University/College : _____
_____

Address of the Institute : _____

: _____

: _____

: _____

_____ _____
Sign of Class/Subject Teacher **Sign of Principal**

_____ _____
Sign of External Examiner **Sign of Internal Examiner**

1. TERMINOLOGIES

Abnormal Behavior

Abnormal behavior describes a person's covert and overt activities that are deviating from the normal behavior. For example, unreasonable fear or intense dislike of an object situation (phobia) or being depressed.

Adjustment

There are different types of changes to which a person has to adjust himself. These changes can be environmental, e.g. change in temperature, humidity and oxygen level; spatial, e.g. change of place and psychosocial, e.g. the husband leaves the job, family members face a problem of change of job of the head of the family.

Adjustment is defined as the series of techniques, methods or processes by which an individual tries to meet the environmental, spatial or psychological changes and maintains a satisfactory equilibrium (balance) with his world. This is also called adaptation.

Sudden death of father is a crisis situation in the family. The wife and children have to adjust to various changes such as financial problem, change of house and feeling of the loss of father. Acceptance of the death of husband, taking up a job to manage the financial problem and continuing the education of children are some of the techniques or methods which the wife may adapt with her world in order to adjust.

Amnesia

Amnesia or absence of memory may be complete, partial, continuous or circumscribed. Complete amnesia for entire previous existence is rare. Retrograde amnesia involves only past events not progressive. Anterograde amnesia involves forgetting the recent event. Circumscribed amnesia involves forgetting the recent event or group of events which usually have strong emotional reasons. Amnesia can be organic, functional or psychogenic.

Anxiety

Anxiety is an unpleasurable reaction to an unreal or imagined danger, whereas fear is a reaction to a real or threatened situation.

Apathy

Apathy is the absence of affect. In apathy, the patient shows indaquate sensitiveness to those experiences that normally give rise to pleasure or pain. The face shows an emptiness of expression. The patient shows lack of interest in all those activities which previously appealed to him. He complains that he cannot respond with any feeling to incidents which should arouse emotions of any kind. It is a symptom of schizophrenia.

Behavior

Behavior means all the covert and overt activities of human beings that can be observed. Behavior may be classified as cognitive, affective and psychomotor. Cognitive refers to knowing, affective refers to feeling and psychomotor relates to doing.

Circumstantiality

In circumstantiality the patient finally reaches his objective but only after many unnecessary or trivial details. He is not able to distinguish essentials from nonessentials. For example, the nurse may ask the patient, "What time did you get up in the morning?" The patient replied, "I went to bed at 9 pm and a neighboring patient disturbed me. I think it was 1 am, I took an apple then I read the Flimfare. After reading it for sometime, I dusted my bed, switched off the light, went to the nurse and said to her "I am going to sleep". So I slept. In the morning, I heard some footsteps but I kept on sleeping, and then you woke me up. I think it is 7 am. So I got up 7 am. The patient beats around the bush and comes to the point at the end.

Déjà vu

It is an illusion of recognition in which a new situation is incorrectly regarded as a repetition of a previous memory. In contrast **Jamais vu** is a feeling of strangeness to familiar situations or events.

Delirium

Delirium is much more than a disturbance of consciousness. It is seen in acute brain syndrome. This syndrome consists of clouding of consciousness, restlessness, confusion, disorientation, illusions and hallucination, apprehension and fear. Delirium occurs in conditions of fever, toxic states, metabolic disturbance like uremia and head trauma.

Delusion

Delusion is defined as a false, fixed unshakable belief, not in accord with one's intelligence, sociocultural and educational background. These are not shared by others. This belief is considered by the viewer as improper or impossible.

Dementia

It is a permanent irreversible loss of intellectual efficiency. It may occur due to structural disturbances or degeneration of the higher cortical neurons due to prolonged toxication or malnutrition. Patients may have a lack of initiativeness, blunting of concern, disorientation, confusion and judgment may be defective. It is seen in organic brain disorders, neoplasms and trauma.

Depression

Depression is the common type of complaint in psychiatric patients. In depression the patient will be quiet, restrained, unhappy and pessimistic. Patient will have a feeling of lassitude, inadequacy, discouragement and hopelessness. His attention and concentration are also impaired due to depressive ramification.

Echolalia

It is the repetition by imitation of speech by another person. In other words, the question is echoed back or repeated. For example, the nurse asks the patient, what is your name? The patient repeats the words "what is your name".

Echopraxia

In echopraxia the activities done by the people are repeated or imitated by the patient.

Ecstasy

In ecstasy the mood is peculiar and peaceful. A religious feeling is the essential part of the state. The patient feels detached from the world and has often a feeling that he is reborn.

Elation

Elation is a joyful affect and is used for sheer happiness. The patient's motor activities and biological drive are increased.

Euphoria

A moderately pleasurable affect is known as euphoria. Here the person gets a feeling of well-being. Person has constant sense of pleasant feeling and is optimistic. Euphoria is seen in hypomanic patients, in certain organic brain disorders and in some cases of frontal lobe tumor.

Exaltation

Exaltation has an element of grandeur along with elation symptoms.

Flight of Ideas

In some of the mental disorders there is disturbance of the stream of thought, thinking processes appear too quickly, the tempo is accelerated. For example, Raja Ram, when asked if he was happy, replied with a rapid flow of thought: "Yes, you have to be cheerful. Flowers are nice and their colors are good. I like his shirt, it is well stitched. I have to look smart". The flight of idea is associated with an increased internal drive. Here the patient is talking and connecting the ideas of happiness with those of smartness.

Sometimes, the rapid flow of thoughts is expressed in words that are similar in sound. The patient uses them in rhythmic war like "Bat Cat Rat Hat Nat Pat Sat Chat." This is known as clang association.

Grief and Mourning

Grief and mourning should be differentiated from depression. Grief is due to loss of close personal association. Grief and mourning are self-limiting and seldom lead to serious important of activities. This may be normal feeling but when persists for a longer duration it becomes a disorder of affect.

Hallucination

Hallucination is perception of a stimulus in the absence of an actual sensory stimulus.

Health

The World Health Organization (WHO) defines 'health' as "a state of complete physical, mental, social and spiritual well-being and not merely the absence of disease or infirmity."

Hypermnesia

Hypermnesia or excessive retention of memories as seen in paranoid psychoses and in manic state, it is limited to a specific period or specific events which may have an emotional factor. So the patient will be able to recall the minute details also of the event or period.

Illusion

Illusion is mistaken or misinterpretation of sense impressions. It means, the clear stimulus has been improperly identified. In the dark, one sees a rope which is misinterpreted as a snake, but on proper illumination the mistake gets corrected. In illusion the object or stimulus is always present which is misinterpreted. Illusion often occurs due to an individual's emotional state, needs and fears.

Insanity

Insanity is a social and legal term. It means that an individual is incompetent to manage his affairs and is not able to foresee the effect of his action. According to the Indian Lunacy Act (Act IV of 1912), a Lunatic or an Idiot is a person of an unsound mind. According to the Mental Health Act 1987, a mentally ill person means a person who is in need of treatment by reason of any mental disorder other than mental retardation. (Chapter I, Clause 2, section (i) Government of India, Ministry of Law and Justice).

Insight

Insight is explained as when the patient is able to understand and realize the significance of his symptoms and of the situation in which he finds himself. When the person is not able to understand about the abnormal behavior which is occurring due to mental disorders and refuses to take treatment, it is said the insight is absent.

Mental Disorder

It includes all the abnormal behavior patterns which range from normal abnormalcy to abnormal abnormalcy. Normal abnormalcy refers to deviating behavior persistently. For example, a girl starts vomiting before the examination. The vomiting stops after the examination is over. In abnormal abnormalcy, the vomiting continues even after the examination is over.

Mental Health

In narrow sense, mental health is described as healthy mind. But it cannot be described without physical, social and spiritual health. Therefore, mental health is a part of general health. It requires a balance between the body, mind and spirit and the environment in which a person lives.

Characteristic of Mentally Healthy Person

- A mentally healthy individual is well adjusted with himself and with society
- A mentally healthy person respects others
- A mentally healthy person is able to solve his problem in a way so that he or she is able to cope or adjust with a crisis or stressful situation with or without minimum assistance of his family and friends.

Mental Illness

Mental illness occurs when a state of physical, mental, social and spiritual wellbeing is disturbed. In illness the individual shows symptoms like depression, felling of anxiety, physical complaints without any organic cause and a sudden change in behavior or mood.

The American Psychiatric Association defines "mental illness or mental disorder as an illness or syndrome with psychological or behavioral manifestations and/or impairment in functioning due to social, psychological, genetic, physical/chemical or biological disturbance. The disorder is not limited to relation between the person and society. The illness is characterized by symptoms and/or impairment in functioning." —APA 1994

Mind

Although mind is not a scientific term, it is used commonly. It is a philosophical term. According to Encyclopedia by Miller and Keane, "Mind the Psyche is the faculty by which one is aware of surroundings and by which one is able to experience emotion, remember, reason and make decision."

In other words, mind is an abstract component which arises out of the central nervous system and develops along with other developments in the human body. It has two components (i) Organic component and (ii) Psychological component, i.e. feeling, emotions, etc.

Mood Swing

It is described as oscillation of mood between two extreme feelings, such as a period euphoria and depression.

Panic

It is a state of extreme, acute, intense anxiety accompanied by disorganization of ego functions.

Paramnesia

Paramnesia is a false re-collection where the patient talks about those events which never took place or gives a false coloring to those that did not happen. For example, in confabulation the patient fills the gap in his memory by fabrications or by making up on his own.

Personality

Personality is the word derived from Latin word Persona meaning person. The dictionary meaning of the word personality is personal existence or identity. According to Taylor, "Personality refers to the aggregate of the physical and mental qualities of the individual as these interact in characteristic fashion with the individual's environment". Personality is expressed through behavior which distinguishes one individual from another. For example, some people are pleasant or unpleasant, some are smart or shabby and some are called quiet or talkative. There are individual characteristic. In unit II of this chapter, personality will be discussed in detail.

Psychiatric Nursing

Psychiatric nursing is the promotion of mental health, prevention of mental illness and care and rehabilitation of a patient with mental illness.

Peplau has defined nursing as a significant, therapeutic interpersonal process that aims to promote a patient's health in the direction of creative, construction, productive and community living. —Peplau, 1952

Psychopathology

- "Phyche" refers to soul or mind, "pathos" traces disease and "logos" means a study. Psychopathology refers to the study of the causes and nature of disease or abnormal behavior.

Suicide

Violence toward self may lead to suicide or an "act of killing oneself". Suicide is commonly seen in depressive patients and at time in schizophrenic patients.

Tangentiality

In this disorders of progression of thought, the patient begins to respond to a question, follow a series of related topics. But he never reaches the goal, unlike in circumstantiality where the patient gives the final answer to the question asked.

Circumstantiality and tangentiality are also known as disorders of direction.

Thought Retardation

In thought retardation the initiation and movement of thought are slow. The patient speaks slowly in a low tone and takes a very long time to complete the answer. Thought retardation is often seen in a depressive phase of manic depressive psychoses. It is also noted sometimes in schizophrenia withdrawn state.

Violences

Violence is an aggressive behavior in which physical force is exerted. Violence is used in war, assassination, murder, assault, rape and even in suicide.

Practical Record Book of Psychiatric Nursing

ORIENTATION

LAYOUT OF MENTAL HEALTH SETTING

ORGANIZATION CHART OF MENTAL HEALTH SETTING

PROCEDURES

1. ADMISSION AND DISCHARGE PROCEDURE

Admission of Mentally Ill Patient

The psychiatric patient can be admitted by the medical officer incharge of the hospital on request even without the application made by the patient. Similarly, the person who is admitted can be discharged within 24 hours. Admission of mentally ill patients can be on:

- Voluntary basis
- Under special circumstances
- Admission by the police officer or magistrate
- **Admission on voluntary basis:** Any person (except a minor) who considers himself to be a mentally ill person and desires to be admitted to any psychiatric hospital or psychiatric nursing home for treatment, may request the medical officer incharge for being admitted on a voluntary basis.

    A minor voluntary patient can be admitted at the request of his/her guardian.

    The patient is admitted for 24 hours. Then a board, consisting of two medical officers, will decide whether such a voluntary patient needs further treatment or should be discharged. In that case the treatment is continued for a period of not exceeding 90 days at a time.

- **Admission under special circumstances:** Any mentally ill person who does not, or is unable to, express his willingness for admission as a voluntary patient, may be admitted or kept as an inpatient in a psychiatric hospital or psychiatric nursing home on an application made by his/her relative or friend. If the medical officer incharge is satisfied that in the interest of the mentally ill person it is necessary to keep him/her under treatment, he/she is kept as an inpatient in the hospital.

    Application on a prescribed form shall be accompanied by two medical certificates from two medical officers, one of whom should be in Government Service. They should explain the condition of the mentally ill patient, such that he should be treated as an inpatient in a psychiatric hospital.

- **Admission by the police officer and magistrate:** A police officer, under Section 23 of the Indian Mental Health Act, 1987, may take into protection any person found wandering within the limits of his station. The officer should have reason to believe that the person is mentally ill and is incapable of taking care of himself. He can be dangerous by reason of his mental illness.

    Such patient is produced before a nearby magistrate within 24 hours of detention.

The magistrate shall:
- Examine the person to assess his capacity to understand.
- Cause him to be examined by a medical officer, and
- Make such inquiries about the person as he may deem necessary.

If the medical officer certifies and the magistrate is satisfied that the person is mentally ill, he is treated as an inpatient in the psychiatric hospital. This is in the interest of the patient's health and personal security.

Discharge of Mentally Ill Patient

The medical officer incharge of a psychiatric hospital or psychiatric nursing home may on the recommendation of two medical practitioners, one of whom shall preferable be a psychiatric, by order in writing, direct the discharge of any person, other than a voluntary patient detained or undergoing treatment as an inpatient. Such a patient should thereupon be discharged from the psychiatric hospital or phychiatric nursing home, provided there is no order from any other authority like the superintendent of prison.

Leave of Absence

Any application for leave or absence on behalf of a mentally ill person (not being a mentally ill prisoner) undergoing treatment as an inpatient in any psychiatric hospital or psychiatric treatment as an inpatient in any psychiatric hospital or psychiatric nursing home may be made to the medical officer incharge.

The application should be submitted duly signed by the relatives who had admitted the patient. It should be accompanied by a bond specifying.

- To take proper care of the mentally ill person.
- To prevent the mentally ill person from causing injury to himself or to other, and
- To bring back the mentally ill to the psychiatric hospital on the expiry of the leave period.
- In case the patient is not brought back after the expiry of the leave period the magistrate needs to be informed.

Format 1

Write the procedure of Admission and Discharge under following heading as:

- Biodata of patient
- Condition of patient at the time of admission
- Type of admission
- Role of nurse at the time of admission

Format 2
Write the procedure of Admission and Discharge under following heading as:
- Biodata of patient
- Condition of patient at the time of admission
- Type of admission
- Role of nurse at the time of admission

Format 3
Write the procedure of Admission and Discharge under following heading as:
- Biodata of patient
- Condition of patient at the time of admission
- Type of admission
- Role of nurse at the time of admission

2. ORTHOSTATIC HYPOTENSION

Introduction

Mild orthostatic hypotension does not need treatment. Many people occasionally feel dizzy or lightheaded after standing and it is usually not causes for concern. The treatment for more—severe cases of orthostatic hypotension depends on the cause. Orthostatic hypotension is often mild, lasting a few seconds to a minutes after standing. However, long lasting orthostatic hypotension can be a sign of more serious.

Definition

Postural hypotension refers to abnormal fall in blood pressure of at least 20 mm Hg in systolic and 10 mm Hg in diastolic and pulse rate will increase by 10–15 beats per minute within three minutes of changing position.

Indication

- Patient having internal or external bleeding
- Patient on diuretic therapy
- Psychiatric patients on antipsychotic drugs may have postural hypotension as a result of side effects.
- Prolonged bed-ridden patients and health elderly above 74 years.

Miscellaneous Indications

- Multiple system atrophy
- Pure autonomic failure
- Autonomic failure associated with Parkinson's disease
- Central nervous system disease
- Peripheral neuropathies
- Systemic disease
- Cardiac impairment
- Old age
- Vasodilation
- Fluid and electrolyte imbalance
- Diabetes

Purpose

- To obtain baseline for diagnosis and treatment.
- To compare with subsequent changes that may occur during care of patient.
- To assist in evaluating status of the patient's blood volume, cardiac output and vascular system.
- To evaluate patient's response to changes in physical condition as are result of treatment with fluids or medications.

Articles

- Sphygmomanometer with adult size cuff
- Stethoscope
- Spirit swab
- Paper bag
- Documentation sheet
- Pen
- Watch

Steps of Procedure

Preprocedural Steps

- Ensure that the patient has been lying down for at least 10 minutes and is relaxed
- Wash your hands to prevent cross-infection
- Check the patient's identification
- Explain the purpose and procedure to the patient as providing information fosters the patient's cooperation and understanding
- Take all the articles to the bedside.

Intraprocedural Steps

- Ask the patient to remove any tight clothing around the arm.
- Before taking initial BP and heart rate measurements, position the patient supine and flat.
- Ensure that the arm is supported at hear level. For example, on a pillow.
- Monitor and count pulse rate for full one minute.
- Select an appropriately sized cuff; its bladder should cover at least 80% of the upper arm but not 100%.
- Clean the stethoscope's ear pieces and diaphragm with a spirit swab to prevent spread of infection.
- Ask the patient to refrain from talking or eating during the procedure as this can result in an inaccurate higher blood pressure measurement being recorded.
- While recording readings, eyes should be parallel to mercury meniscus or number needle. For first baseline reading, inflate the BP cuff and take systolic BP by pulse. For example, if systolic BP is 120 mm Hg then add 40 mm Hg, so that for the next reading if systolic and diastolic BP in supine position raise level up to 160 mm Hg.
- Record and document systolic and diastolic blood pressure and the pulse rate on the documentation chart.
- Teach the patient not to change position suddenly. While getting up from the bed, first take side and gradually get up from bed. Sudden change in position can result in postural change.
- Leaving the cuff in place, ask the patient to sit, ensuring the safety.
- Leaving the cuff in place, allow the patient to stand for 1–3 minutes.
- Ask the patient to walk along the wall so as to avoid sudden fall due to dizziness, if patient experience otherwise no need.
- Check pulse rate in standing position also to see difference between previous and current reading.
- Observer may place the hand under the arm of the client to place it at heart level.
- Place the BP apparatus at heart level with assistance of other nursing personnel.
- Record the BP and document the readings simultaneously to avoid any confusion.
- Note for any change in reading.
- Remove the BP cuff from the arm of the patient.
- Relax and reposition the patient.

Postprocedural Steps

- More all the articles from the bedside to treatment room.
- Mark arrows to denote various position on chart while recording like for supine position mark → and for standing position mark.

Format 1

Write the procedure of orthostatic hypotension under following heading as:
- Biodata of patient
- Steps of procedure
- Observation and recordings
- Role of nurse while doing procedure

Format 2

Write the procedure of orthostatic hypotension under following heading as:
- Biodata of patient
- Steps of procedure
- Observation and recordings
- Role of nurse while doing procedure

Format 3

Write the procedure of orthostatic hypotension under following heading as:
- Biodata of patient
- Steps of procedure
- Observation and recordings
- Role of nurse while doing procedure

3. ORAL MEDICATION

Oral administration is a *route of administration* where a substance is taken through the *mouth*. Per os (PO) is sometimes used as an abbreviation for *medication* to be taken orally. Many medications are taken orally because they are intended to have a *systemic effect*, reaching different parts of the body via the *bloodstream*, for example.

Scope

Oral administration is a part of *enteral administration*, which also includes:
- *Buccal*, dissolved inside the cheek
- *Sublabial*, dissolved under the lip
- *Sublingual administration*, dissolved under the tongue, but due to rapid absorption many consider SL a parenteral route.

Enteral medications come in various forms, including:
- Tablets to swallow, chew or dissolve in water or under the tongue
- Capsules and chewable capsules (with a coating that dissolves in the stomach or bowel to release the medication there)
- Time-release or sustained-release tablets and capsules (which release the medication gradually)
- Powders or granules
- Teas
- Drops
- Liquid medications or syrups

The ten rights of oral medication

The ten 'R's for safe multidisciplinary drug administration—to reduce distractions, consider protected time, the use of a bright tabard or the use of a visual reminder (such as 'do not disturb'), communicating to others that you are not to be interrupted before administration. The ten 'R's consider the following:

- **Right patient**
  - Has this patient been prescribed the drug?
  - Has the patient's name band been checked? Is there a clear patient identifier?
  - Does the patient know he is receiving the drug and why?
- **Right drug**
  - Do you know where to obtain the drug? Are all drugs in one location and are they clearly labeled?
  - Is this the drug that has been prescribed? Is there a drug with a similar name?

  If appropriate, has the drug been checked by another nurse or health professional?
- **Right dosage**
  - Is the dose appropriate or usual for the drug being prescribed?
  - If appropriate, has the dose or calculation been checked by another nurse or health professional?
- **Right time**
  - Has the time gap between each drug administration been adequate, sufficient, too short or too long?
- **Right route**
  - Is the route appropriate for the drug being prescribed?
- **Right to refuse** (patient and nurse)
  - Are you able to exercise your clinical judgment and refuse to give or omit the drug? Do you have a rationale for this and are you able to demonstrate or explain this to others?
  - Do you know what action to take if the patient refuses the prescribed medication?
  - Can you identify the barriers to medication administration and identify suitable approaches to address them (dysphagia or confusion, for example) immediately before administration?
- **Right knowledge**
  - Do you know what monitoring is required prior to administration?

- Do you know how to prepare and administer the medication in line with local policies?
- Do you know the preferences of the patient?
- Do you understand the pharmacokinetics, pharmacodynamics, action, possible interactions, side-effects, expected positive outcome(s), and/or the possible occurrence of adverse effects (toxicity), or overdose of the drug(s) you are administering?
- Do you understand the law related to the particular drug(s)?

☐ **Right questions or challenges**
- Is this the right prescription, appropriate drug(s) for the patient's condition(s)? Is the prescription written correctly and clearly, with clear unambiguous instructions?
- Can the writing be easily read?
- Can you communicate with other professionals if needed?
- Is there access to available resources (drug formularies and/or product information leaflets)?

☐ **Right advice**
- Does the patient know about the drug? If not, can you give the patient advice/details/information about this/these medication(s)?

☐ **Right response or outcome**
- Do you know the expected response/outcomes of the drug?
- Do you know how to observe/check for allergic reactions, drug interaction(s), side-effects and call for assistance?
- Do you know how and when to complete records of administration in line with local policy and document any changes?

Steps of Oral Medication Procedure

☐ Gather equipment. Check each medication order against original physician's order according to agency policy. Clarify any inconsistencies. Check patient's chart for allergies.
☐ Know actions, special nursing consideration, and adverse effects of medications to be administered.
☐ Perform proper hand hygiene.
☐ Move medication cart outside patient's room or prepare for administration in medication area.
☐ Unlock medication cart or drawer.
☐ Prepare medications for one patient at a time.
☐ Select proper medication from drawer or stock and compare with drug sheet. Check expiration dates and perform calculations, if necessary.
☐ Place unit dose-package medications in a disposable cup. Do not open wrapper until at bedside. Keep narcotics and medications that require special nursing assessments in a separate container.
☐ When removing tablets or capsules from a bottle, pour the necessary number into bottle cap and then place tablets in a medication cup. Break only scored tablets, if necessary, to obtain proper dose.
☐ Hold liquid medication bottles with the label against palm. Use appropriate measuring device when pouring liquids and read the amount of medication at the bottom of the meniscus at eye level. Wipe bottle lip with a paper towel.
☐ Recheck each medication package or preparation with the order as it is poured.
☐ When all medications for one patient have been prepared, recheck once again with the medication order before taking them to patient.
☐ Carefully transport medications to patient's bedside. Keep medications in sight at all times.
☐ See that patient receives medications at the correct time.
☐ Identify the patient carefully. There are three correct ways to do this
- Check name on patient's identification bracelet.
- Ask patient his or her name.
- Verify patient's identification with a staff member who knows patient.

☐ Complete necessary assessments before administration of medications. Check allergy bracelet or ask patient about allergies. Explain purpose and action of each medication to patient.

- ☐ Assist patient to an upright or lateral position.
- ☐ Administer medications.
  - Offer water or other permitted fluids with pills, capsules, tablets, and some liquid medications.
  - Ask patient's preference regarding medications to be taken by hand or in cup and one at a time or all at once.
  - If capsule or tablet falls to the floor, discard it and administer a new one.
  - Record and fluid intake I-O measurement is ordered.
- ☐ Remain with patient until each medication is swallowed.
- ☐ Perform hand hygiene.
- ☐ Record each medication given on medication chart or record using required format.
  - If drug was refused or omitted, record this in appropriate area on medication record.
  - Recording of administration of a narcotic may require additional documentation on a narcotic record stating drug count and other specific information.
- ☐ Check on patient within 30 minutes of drug administration to verify response to medication.

Format 1

Write the procedure of oral medication under following heading as:

- Biodata of patient
- Steps of procedure
- Observation and recordings
- Role of nurse while doing procedure
- Drug sheet

Format 2

Write the procedure of oral medication under following heading as:
- Biodata of patient
- Steps of procedure
- Observation and recordings
- Role of nurse while doing procedure
- Drug sheet

Format 3

Write the procedure of oral medication under following heading as:

- ☐ Biodata of patient
- ☐ Steps of procedure
- ☐ Observation and recordings
- ☐ Role of nurse while doing procedure
- ☐ Drug sheet

4. ELECTROCONVULSIVE THERAPY (ECT)

Definition

ECT is an artificial induction of a grand mal seizure *through the application* of electrical current to the brain. The stimulus is applied through electrodes that are placed either bilaterally in the frontotemporal region or unilaterally on the non-dominant side.

History

ECT was first performed by Italian psychiatrists Ugo Cerletti and Lucio Bini in Rome in the April 1938.

Parameters of Electrical Current Applied

Standard dose according to American Psychiatric Association, 1978:
- **Voltage:** 70–120 volts
- **Duration:** 0.7–1.5 seconds

Types of Seizure Produced

- **Grand mal seizure:** Tonic phase lasting for 10–15 seconds
- **Clonic phase lasting for** 30–60 seconds

Mechanism of Action

The exact mechanism of action is not known. Only hypothersis states that ECT possibly affects the catecholamine pathways between diencephalon and limbic system also involving the hypothalamus.

Types

- **Direct ECT:** In this, ECT is given in the absence of anesthesia and muscular relaxation. This is not commonly used method now.
- **Modified ECT:** Here ECT is modified by drug-induced muscular relaxation and general anesthesia.

Frequency and Total Number of ECT

- **Frequency:** Three time per week or as indicated
- **Total number:** 6–10; up to 25 or more may be preferred as per severity of the patient's condition and as per indications from doctor.

Applications of Electrodes

- **Bilateral ECT:** Each electrode is placed 2.5–4 cm above the midpoint, on a line joining the tragus of ear and the lateral canthus of the eye.
- **Unilateral ECT:** Electrodes are placed only one side of head, usually nondominant side.

Indications

I. **Major depression:** With suicidal risk, stupor, poor intake of food and fluid, melancholia with psychotic features, unsatisfactory response to drugs or when drugs are contraindicated or have serious side effects.
II. **Severe catatonia:** With stupor, poor intake of food and fluid, melancholia with psychotic features, unsatisfactory response to drugs or when drugs are contraindicated or have serious side effects.

III. **Severe psychosis (schizophrenia or mania):** With risk of suicide, homicide or danger of physical assault, depressive features, unsatisfactory response to drugs or when drug are contraindicated.

IV. **Organic mental disorder**
- Organic mood disorder
- **Organic psychosis**

Contraindication

I. **Absolute**
- **Raised** ICP (Intracranial pressure)

II. **Relatives**
- Cerebral aneurysm
- Cerebral hemorrhage
- Brain tumor
- Acute myocardial infraction
- Congestive heart failure
- Pneumonia
- Retinal detachment

Complications

- Life-threatening complications of ECT are rare.
- Fracture can sometimes occur in elderly with osteoporosis.

Side Effects

- Memory loss
- Drowsiness, confusion, restlessness
- Poor concentration
- Unsteady gait
- Headache, weakness/fatigue, backache
- Dryness of mouth, nausea, vomiting
- Tongue bite

ECT Team

- Psychiatrist
- Anesthesiologist
- Trained nurse
- Other helper

Preparation of Articles

Resuscitation tray
- Endotracheal tube of different size
- Oral airway of different sizes
- Laryngoscope with blades of different sizes (check for bulb and batteries)
- Facemasks of different sizes
- Magill forceps
- Ambu bag

Emergency medications
- ☐ Inj. Atropine
- ☐ Inj. Adrenaline
- ☐ Inj. Avil
- ☐ Inj. Calcium gluconate
- ☐ Inj. Dopamine
- ☐ Inj. Dexamethasone
- ☐ Inj. Esmolol
- ☐ Inj. Hydrocortisone
- ☐ Inj. KCL
- ☐ Inj. Lorazepam
- ☐ Inj. Lasix
- ☐ Inj. Phenytoin
- ☐ Inj. Sodium bicarbonate

Injection tray
- ☐ Inj. Atropine
- ☐ Inj. Thiopentone
- ☐ Inj. Succinylcholine

Other
- ☐ Bedsheet on ECT table
- ☐ Draw sheet
- ☐ Biomedical waste buckets
- ☐ Defibrillator
- ☐ Cardiac monitor
- ☐ BP apparatus
- ☐ BP cuff and pulse oximetry
- ☐ ECT machine
- ☐ Boyle's apparatus
- ☐ Oxygen cylinder
- ☐ Tongue depressor
- ☐ Mouth gag
- ☐ Suction machine
- ☐ Suction catheter
- ☐ Bowl of water
- ☐ Gloves
- ☐ EEG, ECG
- ☐ Cotton swab for EEG electrodes
- ☐ Jelly for EEG electrodes
- ☐ Jelly for ECG electrodes
- ☐ Jelly for ECT electrodes
- ☐ IV stand and cannula
- ☐ Infusion set
- ☐ Normal saline
- ☐ Syringes
- ☐ Ampoule cutter
- ☐ Spirit swab
- ☐ Kidney tray

Role of Nurse

Preprocedural Steps

- Make patient comfortable and give reassurance and provide supine position.
- Check vital sign and record on vital chart.
- Apply ECG, EEG, ECT electrodes with jelly.
- Start IV line (Normal saline)

Intraprocedural Steps

- Administer inj. Glycopyrrolate (0.2 mg), Atropine (0.65 mg)
- Administer inj. Thiopentone after hyperventilating the patient.
- Apply another BP cuff on the other arm and inflate cuff till 200–250 mm Hg with lock and check pulse.
- Administer inj. Succinylcholine (0.75–1.5 mg/kg body weight).
- Since the muscle relaxant paralyzes all muscle including respiratory muscle, patient airway should be ensured and ventilator support should be started.
- Insert mouth gag to prevent possible tongue bite.
- Monitor voltage, intensity and duration of electrical stimulus given.
- Record duration of seizures after passing current using cuff method.
- Hundred percent oxygen should be provided.
- Check whether seizure duration is adequate (at least 15 seconds of motor seizure)
- During seizure, monitor vital sign, ECG, EEG and oxygen saturation.
- Deflate BP cuff
- Check for any immediate side effect of ECT.
- Record if any emergency medication is given.
- Check and record vital sign.

Postprocedural Steps

- Remove electrode and clean the patient.
- Remove mouth gag.
- Provide suctioning, if necessary.
- Inspect patient's mouth for any injury.
- Check and record vital sign.
- Assess the patient's level of consciousness
- Shift the patient in post ECT room.
- Place the patient in lateral position.
- Provide side rail to prevent fall and injury.
- Continue IV fluid.
- Check and record vital sign on vital chart every 15 minutes for half an hour and once in every 30 minutes till the patient recover to normal stage.
- Check patient status, checking gag reflex, checking orientation, asking for headache, giddiness, assess postictal confusion and restlessness.
- Give reassurance to family member.
- Remove IV cannula when patient starts accepting orally.
- Check for immediate post-ECT side effect.
- Complete the documentation.
- Conduct mini mental state examination (MMSE) once the patient reestablishes to routine self.

Format 1
Write the procedure of ECT under following heading as:
- Biodata of patient
- Steps of procedure
- Observation and recordings
- Role of nurse while doing procedure

Format 2

Write the procedure of ECT under following heading as:

- ☐ Biodata of patient
- ☐ Steps of procedure
- ☐ Observation and recordings
- ☐ Role of nurse while doing procedure

Format 3

Write the procedure of ECT under following heading as:

- Biodata of patient
- Steps of procedure
- Observation and recordings
- Role of nurse while doing procedure

5. RESTRAINING

Introduction

Restraints and seclusion may be required for a patient with a variety of settings including patient with psychiatric illnesses or altered status that become violent and dangerous and pose serious threat to themselves or others.

Definition

Verbal restraining: It is a procedure of using firm and consistent voice to control the undesirable behavior of the patient.
Seclusion: It is a involuntary confinement of a person in specially constructed, locked room equipped with a security window for direct visual monitoring.
Physical restraint: It is a procedure with which a person uses his or her body effectively and immediately control or immobilize another.
- **Manual restraint:** It involves physical force by mental health team to control undesired behavior of the patient.
- **Mechanical restraint:** They are device, usually ankle and wrist restraint, fastened to the bed frame to curtail the patient's physical aggression such as hitting, kicking and hair pulling.

Chemical restraining: It includes use of certain psychopharmacological agents to calm down the aggressive patient. It includes sedatives, antianxiety drugs and antipsychotic drugs.

Indication

- When patient poses threat or harm to self or other.
- Violent acts and behavior.
- Anger and agitated patient.
- All interventions failed to control the behavior.

Contraindication

- Osteomalacia
- Osteoporosis
- Fractures
- Respiratory depression
- ICP
- DM, hypertension and other severe metabolic disorder.

Guiding Principles

- It should not for the comfort of the nursing staff.
- Use the least restrictive to the most restrictive approach.
- Restraints should be applied according to the specific treatment center.
- There should be enough manpower, resources and infrastructure.
- A physician assessment followed by a written order is required specifying type of physical restraint, reason, circumstances for use, duration and condition for discontinuation.
- Neck restraint or metallic restraint should be avoided.
- The attending physician in consultation with the interdisciplinary team members decides to use restraint or seclusion methods.
- In emergency situations, the ward incharge can order for using restraint or seclusion while awaiting the physician's order.
- The reason for using physical restraint or seclusion should be explained to the patient or family.
- The nurse should do continued clinical assessment and evaluation in consultation with physician.
- The nurse should monitor and document the use of restraint or seclusion including the evaluation of the outcome.

Articles: (For Physical Restraint)

- A clean tray containing (for physical restraint)
- Physical restraint made from bandage
- Cotton pads
- Documentation sheet

A Clean Tray Containing (for Chemical Restraint)

- Syringe and needles of different sizes
- Spirit swab: To prepare skin prior to procedure
- Prescribed medications
- Medicine card: To prevent from errors of medicine administration.
- Documentation sheet
- Tray for checking vital signs

I. Verbal De-escalation

- It is the first method of controlling the patient's behavior
- The nurse or the treating team should make every attempt not to aggravate or worsen pre-existing injuries or medical conditions.
- Attempt to control the patient with verbal counseling.

Verbal De-escalation Procedure

When working with agitated patient, there are four main objectives:
- Ensure the safety of the patient, staff and other in this area
- Help the patient, manage his emotions and distress and maintain or regain control of his behavior
- Avoid the use of restraint when at all possible
- Avoid coercive intervention that escalate agitation.

GUIDELINES FOR ENVIRONMENT AND PEOPLE PREPARATION

- Physical space should be designed for safety
- Staff should be appropriate for the job.
- Staff must be adequately
- An adequate number of trained staff must be available.
- Use objective scales to assess agitation.
- Clinician should self-monitor and feel safe when approaching the patient.

10 Domains of De-escalation to Take Care of Agitated Patients

- Respect personal space
- Do not be provocative
- Establish verbal contact
- Be concise
- Identify wants and feelings
- Listen wants and feeling
- Agree or agree to disagree
- Lay down the law and set clear limits

- Offer choices and optimism
- Debrief the patient and staff.

II. SECLUSION GUIDELINES

- The goal is to give the patient the opportunity to regain physical and emotional self-control
- Seclusion decreases stimulation, protects others from the patient, prevent property out
- The seclusion room should be near to the nursing station
- For safety the room, wall and floor should be well padded
- Any sharp or potentially objects such as pens, glasses, belts, furniture and matches are removed from the patient as safety precaution
- Ceiling fan should be at an appropriate height.
- Electrical sockets should be covered
- There should be one observation window ideally to observe the behavior and to provide food to the patient.
- Patient should be monitored every 15 minutes.

Steps of Procedure

Preprocedural Steps

- Assess and observe violent acts and behavior of agitated patients.
- Take written order from concerned psychiatric in instruction book for secluding the patient
- Check physical set-up for seclusion room.

Intraprocedural Steps

- Take help from other nursing personnel to control agitated patients
- Bring agitated patient to meet nutritional and elimination needs
- Make observations for behavior intermittently for further intervention.

Postprocedural Steps

- Record and report about current behavior of patient to the concerned psychiatrist
- If needed, receive further order or renewal for controlling patient.

III. PHYSICAL RESTRAINTS

Physical Restraint Procedure

- Use the minimum physical restraint required to accomplish necessary patient care and ensure safe transportation.
- Ensure sufficient personnel. 4–6 trained staff members are needed to restrain as aggressive patient safety.
- The patient is informed that his or her behavior is out of control and that the staff are taking control to provide safety and prevent injury.
- **One person approach:** The patient is approached from back and the nurse restricts the movement of patient by blocking the movement of shoulder joint and neck by making knot with both wrists at the back of patient's neck.
- **Two persons approach:** The patient is approached from front and each nurse restricts movement by grabbing each hand and restricting the arm and shoulder joint.
- Patient is dragged toward the back keeping in mind the safety of the patient.
- Four staff members each take a limb.

- The patient is transported by stretcher or carried to a seclusion room, and restraints are applied to each limb and fastened to the bed frame and not to the railings.
- Place padding under patient's head and under restraint to prevent the patient's from further harming him/himself.
- Document circulatory status, cyanosis and ecchymosis, edema and eruption of restrained extremities.
- Take vital sign every 15 minutes.

Mechanical Approach

- It involves applying device such as rope or a rolled long cloth along with sufficient padding in order to restrict the movement.
- This approach can be used by making a clove hitch knot or a figure-of-eight knot.
- Since clove hitch knot is more preferred because of less injury to the skin.

Removal of Restraints

Guidelines

- As soon as possible, staff members must inform the patient of the behavioral criteria that will be used to determine whether to decrease or to end the use of restraint or seclusion.
- Encourage the patient to talk about the situation that led to the aggressive behavior.

Procedure

- Remove restraint gradually
- Monitor patient's response to removal of restraint and assess the pressure area keenly.
- Discuss all components of the incident with the patient.
- Avoid asking humiliating questions.

IV. CHEMICAL RESTRAINTS

Procedure

- Assess the need for chemical restraining and use only when other two methods are failed.
- Have sedatives medication prepared for injection.
- Assess the need for sedatives carefully and keep the antidote in case of over dosage.
- Monitor for side effect of the drug.
- Monitor vital sign for assessing possible side effect of the drug.

Documentation

- Biodata of the patient.
- Nature of the patient's violence and record patient's comments verbatim.
- Use of other techniques for avoiding the use of restraints.
- Reason for restraints.
- Physician who provided the order.
- Kind of restraint used.
- Patient's response to treatment.
- Nursing care provided throughout the intervention.
- Rationale for termination of the procedure.

Format 1

Write the procedure of Restraining under following heading as:

- ☐ Biodata of patient
- ☐ Indications for restraining
- ☐ Types of restraints for patient
- ☐ Role of nurse while doing procedure
- ☐ Observation and recordings after restraining

Format 2

Write the procedure of Restraining under following heading as:

- Biodata of patient
- Indications for restraining
- Types of restraints for patient
- Role of nurse while doing procedure
- Observation and recordings after restraining

Format 3

Write the procedure of Restraining under following heading as:
- Biodata of patient
- Indications for restraining
- Types of restraints for patient
- Role of nurse while doing procedure
- Observation and recordings after restraining

EXAMPLE OF HISTORY TAKING

INTRODUCTION

It is the important part of psychiatric examination. A good history help considerably to make psychiatric diagnosis and treatment plans. Most of the psychiatry illnesses are the end result of a series of traumatic life experiences a person goes through from the early childhood.

PURPOSE

To understand the drawback in personality of individual and his present illness.

One should try to gather information from all possible sources. One should interview each attendant separately and their account should be kept separately. If patient has come alone in the first visit, he should be advised to bring one of the close family members in the next visit to get more information. Both patient and his attendant's need to be taken in confidence that information given by them would be kept strictly confidential.

Points to be Kept in Mind while Taking History

- Nurse should express keen interest in patient's problems.
- One should not give an impression that she is in hurry.
- Interpretation should be minimal especially in the early part of history taking.
- Do not take any person for his illness and not to take side of patient or of his relatives. Always should try to have a neutral approach.
- Try to avoid too much exploration in the first interview. It may increase anxiety of the patient and he may become uncooperative.
- Keenly observe interaction between patient and his relatives.
- Nurse should look like more as a friend and a guide, who is interested in the problem of patient. One should not give an impression as if one is like a detective.
- Try to gather information from all possible sources.

IDENTIFICATION DATA

Name: _____   Age: _____

Sex: _____   CR no: _____

Address: _____   Bed no: _____

Marital status: _____   Religion: _____

Education: _____   Occupation: _____

Income: _____   DOA: _____

Informants

Sometime the history provided by a psychiatric patient may be incomplete, due to factors like absent insight or uncooperativeness, it is important to take the history from the patient's relatives who are acting as informants. Mention here:

- Source of information
- Relation of the informant to patient
- Intimacy and length of acquaintance with patient
- Reliability of information

Note:
- In psychotic illness, relatives will be able to provide more reliable information
- In neurotic illness, patient would be the best informant.

CHIEF COMPLAINTS

(Why patient has come or been brought in hospital)

The chief complaint is recorded in patient's own words. The patient's explanation should be recorded as verbatim (patient's version). Record the informant's version separately. If the patient says that he has no complaints, this should also recorded. Try to write in a chronological order.
- **According to patient (Observe behavior)**
  Complaint (patient's verbatim) x duration
- **According to relatives (observe behavior)**
  Complaint (relative's version) x duration

Note: Keen observation must be there to correlate the overt Behavior of the patient with provided information.

HISTORY OF PRESENT ILLNESS

It provides a comprehensive and chronological picture of the events leading up to the current moment in the patient's life. History of present illness is the most helpful in making a diagnosis.
- **Onset:** onset of symptoms is
  - Abrupt (within 24 hrs)
  - Acute (within 2 wks)
  - Sub-acute (more than 2 wks)
  - Insidious (More than 4 wks)
- **Precipitating Factors:** Enquire about any precipitating events. These could be:
  - Physical e.g. a febrile illness
  - Psychological e.g. death/loss, stressful event in life

  Note: Ascertain whether the events clearly preceded the illness or were consequences of the illness. E.g. job loss following onset of Schizophrenia.
- **Course of illness:** The course of illness can be:
  - Episodic – discrete symptomatic period with intervening periods of normalcy
  - Continuous or fluctuating – Periodic exacerbations of a continuous illness
- **Associated disturbances:** Enquiry should also be made of impairment in other areas of functioning these include:
  - Disturbances in sleep
  - Disturbances in appetite
  - Disturbances in weight
  - Disturbances in sexual life
  - Disturbances in social life
  - Disturbances in occupational life

  Note: Specify the nature of disturbance
- **Rule out any organic etiology, ask about**
  History of trauma, fever, headache, vomiting, confusion, substance abuse

  Note: Enquire about the presence of suicidal ideation

Pattern of writing history of present illness as follows:

Patient was apparently well before 6 months. After this, family members noticed a sudden change in the Behavior of patient in form of decreased interaction with family members, being sad and refusal to take food. From last 1 month, patient was not doing any work and staying in his room for the whole day. Three days back, Patient attempts to commit suicide by hanging himself to the ceiling, but he was saved by her elder brother.

PAST HISTORY

History of similar or any other psychiatric illness in the past.
Medical History: H/O hypertension, coronary artery disease, accidents, diabetes mellitus, convulsions and related hospitalization.
Surgical History: H/O of surgical procedures

Psychiatric History

- H/O past psychiatric episodes with symptoms & Behavior
- Description of psychiatric hospitalization (with name of hospital)
- H/O alcohol & drug abuse or dependence
- Description of psychiatric medications took in past
- Number of ECTs received (If given)

Note: Write psychiatric history in chronological order.

FAMILY HISTORY

- **Draw family tree**
- **Give a description of the individual family members (parents & siblings)**

Parents (Patient's Father and Mother)

- Age of parents (if dead, write age at the time of death and cause of death, write age of patient at the time of mother's death)
- Health status
- Education
- Occupation
- Emotional bonding with patient

Pattern of writing as follows:
Patient's father is 68 yrs old, healthy, educated up to 8th standard, doing farming and he is emotionally attached to patient's elder brother whereas bonding with patient is less.

Patient's mother is 64 yrs old, unhealthy (hypertensive since 2008 and taking medication atenolol 5 mg/day), educated up to 8th standard, homemaker. She has strong emotional bonding with patient.

Siblings (Patient's Brother and Sister)

- Write in chronological order of birth with name & age
- Marital status
- Education
- Occupation
- Health
- Emotional bonding with patient

Pattern of writing as follows:
Patient has one elder brother who is 35 yrs old, educated up to B.A, married, doing job in factory, healthy and he is not much attached with patient.

Patient has one younger sister who is 25 yrs, educated up to 10th standard, unmarried, staying at home, healthy and she has strong emotional bonding with patient.

General Background of Family

- ☐ Joint or nuclear family
- ☐ Social status
- ☐ Detail of mental illness in family
- ☐ Detail of physical illness in family
- ☐ Detail of interpersonal relationship among family members

Pattern of writing

Patient belongs to nuclear middle class family, no history of any physical and mental illness in patient's family. There is good interpersonal relationship among all the family members.

PERSONAL HISTORY

Birth and Early Development

Enquire about the following:
- ☐ Patient was a wanted/unwanted child
- ☐ Born at full term or premature
- ☐ Cry immediate or delayed
- ☐ Weight at the time of birth
- ☐ Date of time and birth
- ☐ Delivered in hospital or at home (by trained person or not)
- ☐ Any complications during delivery
- ☐ Type of delivery (normal or LSCS)
- ☐ Type of feeding (breast feeding or bottle feeding). Also mention the duration of exclusive breast feeding
- ☐ Age of starting weaning diet with feeding difficulties
- ☐ Mother-child bonding
- ☐ Care taker of child at home (mother, grand mother or any other person)
- ☐ Mention development milestones in accordance to age (delayed/early/normal)
- ☐ Type of toilet training (strict or lenient)

Pattern of writing

Patient was a wanted child, born in 1990 at full term in hospital by normal delivery which was done by Gynecologist, patient cried immediately after birth and weight of patient was 3.4 kg at birth. no H/O of any complication during delivery. Patient was on exclusive breast feeding for 4 months after this weaning diet was started at the age of 4 months. Mother did not find any difficulty in starting weaning diet. Mother was strongly attached to patient as she was taking care of patient at home. Patient started sitting at the age of 6 months, standing with support at 8 months, standing without support at 9 months, walking at 1 yr, uttering voices at 8 months and speaking at 1 yr, running at 1 1/2 yr. thus all the developmental milestones were found to be normal according to age. Toilet training was given at the age of 2-3 yrs by mother and it was normal.

Behavior During Childhood

- ☐ Enquire about sleep disturbances such as night mares, night terrors, sleep walking
- ☐ Presence of neurotic traits such as thumb sucking, nail biting, temper tantrums, bed wetting (enuresis), encopresis, stammering, presence of tics.
- ☐ Look for conduct disturbances in the form of frequent fights, truancy, stealing, lying, gang activities
- ☐ Enquire about relationship with parents, siblings and peers

Physical Illness During Childhood

- Record physical illness suffered in childhood.
- Enquire specially regarding epilepsy, meningitis and encephalitis

School Record

- Age of beginning and finishing education (Govt/Private/Convent)
- Location of school (rural or urban)
- Standard reached
- Academic achievements
- Relationship with teachers and peers (Nicknames by friends)
- Attitude to home work
- Reason for termination of studies (if occur prematurely)
- Any learning difficulties
- Number of friends in school
- If not attended school give reasons, disadvantages, dissatisfaction or anxiety caused by illiteracy.

Pattern of writing

Patient started his schooling at the age of 4 yrs, he joined private school located in rural area. He had 5-6 friends in school. He was educated up to 10th standard and after that he terminated his study because of lack of interest in studies. He was an average student and had good relationship with teachers and peer group. He experienced learning difficulties in the form of forgetfulness.

Occupational Record

- Age of starting work
- Jobs held in chronological order (how long held)
- Reasons for job changes
- Job satisfaction
- Relationship with authorities and colleagues

Pattern of writing

Patient started doing job at the age of 24 yrs. He used to changed his jobs frequently after every 5-6 months) because of lack of interest in doing job. He was not satisfied with Behavior of his boss and other colleagues. He did not like interact with his colleagues much.

Play History

- Indoor/outdoor games, with whom (friends or siblings)
- Solitary play
- Sharing of toys with siblings/friends

Menstrual History (In Case of Female Patient)

- Age of menarche
- Reaction to menarche
- Regularity of periods
- Duration of menses
- Presence of dysmenorrhoea/menorrhagia/oligomenorrhea
- Emotional disturbances in relation to menstrual cycle

Sexual History

Question should be asked in a free and frank manner, but patient's personal information must be respected. Social & cultural background of the patient must be kept in mind.
- Sexual information (how acquired)
- Patient's attitude towards sex education
- In male patient–guilt and sexual fantasies associated with it, homosexuality or any other sexual perversions
- Heterosexual experiences apart from marriage

Marital History

- Married/unmarried
- Type of marriage (Love or arrange)
- Duration of marriage
- Interpersonal relations
- Number of children
- Contraceptive measure
- Termination of pregnancy if any

Practical Record Book of Psychiatric Nursing

FORMAT OF HISTORY TAKING/COLLECTION

Format 1

BIODATA

Name: _____ Age: _____
Sex: _____ Address: _____
Education: _____ Occupation: _____
Marital status: _____ Religion: _____
Socioeconomic status: _____ Informant: _____
Reliability of informant: _____

Informants

_____
_____
_____

CHIEF COMPLAINTS

_____
_____
_____
_____
_____
_____
_____

According to Patient

_____
_____
_____
_____
_____
_____
_____

According to Relatives/Records

History of Present Illness

Past History

Past Psychiatric and Medical History

Family History

Family Tree

PERSONAL HISTORY

Birth and Development

Behaviour During Childhood

Physical Illness during Childhood

School record

Occupational record

Play history

Menstrual history (In case of female patient)

Sexual history

Marital history

PREMORBID PERSONALITY

Interpersonal Relationship

Use of Leisure Time

Premorbid Mood

Attitude Towards Self and Others

Attitude Towards Work and Responsibility

Religious Belief

Fantasy Life

Habits

INFERENCE OF HISTORY TAKING

FORMAT OF HISTORY TAKING/COLLECTION

Format 2

IDENTIFICATION DATA

Name: _____ Age: _____
Sex: _____ Address: _____
Education: _____ Occupation: _____
Marital status: _____ Religion: _____
Socioeconomic status: _____ Informant: _____
Reliability of informant: _____

Chief Complaints

_____
_____
_____
_____
_____
_____
_____
_____
_____
_____
_____

According to Patient

_____
_____
_____
_____
_____
_____
_____
_____
_____
_____
_____
_____

According to Relatives/Records

Present Illness

Past psychiatric and Medical History

Family History

_____
_____
_____
_____
_____
_____
_____

Family Tree

Prenatal History

Birth History

Childhood History

Educational History

Play History

Puberty

Occupational History

Sexual and Marital History

Premorbid Personality

Interpersonal Relationship

Use of Leisure Time

Premorbid Mood

Attitude Towards Self and Others

Attitude Towards Work and Responsibility

Religious Belief

Fantasy Life

Habits

Inference of History Taking

Practical Record Book of Psychiatric Nursing

FORMAT OF HISTORY TAKING/COLLECTION

Format 3

BIODATA

Name: _____ Age: _____
Sex: _____ Address: _____
Education: _____ Occupation: _____
Marital status: _____ Religion: _____
Socioeconomic status: _____ Informant: _____
Reliability of informant: _____

Chief Complaints

_____
_____
_____
_____
_____
_____
_____
_____
_____
_____

According to Patient

_____
_____
_____
_____
_____
_____
_____
_____
_____
_____

According to Relatives/Records

Present Illness

Past psychiatric and Medical History

Family History

___

Family Tree

Prenatal History

___

Birth History

___

Childhood History

___

Educational History

___

Play History

Puberty

Occupational History

Sexual and Marital History

Premorbid Personality

Interpersonal Relationship

_____
_____
_____
_____
_____

Use of Leisure Time

_____
_____
_____
_____
_____

Premorbid Mood

_____
_____
_____
_____
_____

Attitude Towards Self and others

_____
_____
_____
_____
_____

Attitude Towards Work and Responsibility

_____
_____
_____
_____

Religious Belief

Fantasy Life

Habits

Inference of History Taking

FORMAT OF HISTORY TAKING/COLLECTION

Format 4

BIODATA

Name: _____ Age: _____
Sex: _____ Address: _____
Education: _____ Occupation: _____
Marital status: _____ Religion: _____
Socioeconomic status: _____ Informant: _____
Reliability of informant: _____

Chief Complaints

_____
_____
_____
_____
_____
_____
_____
_____
_____
_____

According to Patient

_____
_____
_____
_____
_____
_____
_____
_____
_____
_____

According to Relatives/Records

Present Illness

Past psychiatric and Medical History

Family History

Family Tree

Prenatal History

Birth History

Childhood History

Educational History

Play History

___

Puberty

___

Occupational History

___

Sexual and Marital History

___

Premorbid Personality

___

Interpersonal Relationship

_____
_____
_____
_____
_____

Use of Leisure Time

_____
_____
_____
_____
_____

Premorbid Mood

_____
_____
_____
_____
_____

Attitude Towards Self and others

_____
_____
_____
_____
_____

Attitude Towards Work and Responsibility

_____
_____
_____
_____
_____

Religious Belief

Fantasy Life

Habits

Inference of History Taking

Practical Record Book of Psychiatric Nursing

FORMAT OF HISTORY TAKING/COLLECTION

Format 5

BIODATA

Name: _____ Age: _____
Sex: _____ Address: _____
Education: _____ Occupation: _____
Marital status: _____ Religion: _____
Socioeconomic status: _____ Informant: _____
Reliability of informant: _____

Chief Complaints

_____
_____
_____
_____
_____
_____
_____
_____
_____
_____

According to Patient

_____
_____
_____
_____
_____
_____
_____
_____
_____

According to Relatives/Records

Present Illness

Past psychiatric and Medical History

Family History

Family Tree

Prenatal History

Birth History

Childhood History

Educational History

Play History

Puberty

Occupational History

Sexual and Marital History

Premorbid Personality

Interpersonal Relationship

Use of Leisure Time

Premorbid Mood

Attitude Towards Self and others

Attitude Towards Work and Responsibility

Religious Belief

Fantasy Life

Habits

Inference of History Taking

EXAMPLE OF MENTAL STATUS EXAMINATION

A systematically conducted mental status examination is an important component of case taking it is essential or records the observations properly. Whenever positive findings are obtained, they should be described in detail. It is not adequate to say 'delusions present' or 'hallucinations'. MSE has to be repeated several times during the course of the illness to know the evolution of symptoms, effectiveness of treatment etc. The time frame covered by the MSE restricted to the hour of observation, but extends longer the following account highlights the major components of MSE, details should be obtained from other sources cited.

The mental status examination is a structured assessment of the patient's behavioral and cognitive functioning.

A. GENERAL APPEARANCE (OBSERVATION)

Description as complete, accurate, life like as possible, of the observations of ward staff and your own the following points may be considered, though not exclusively.

- Is the patient co-operative?
- Can adequate rapport be established?
- Does the patient maintain adequate eye contact?
- Facial expression
    - Is it appropriate to and consistent with the subject under discussion?
    - Did it change appropriately with change of subject?
    - Was the patient's face unexpressive and flat?
    - Did he look to be normal attentive, apathetic or indifferent?
    - Did the patient at any time show elation (mild pleasure), appropriate smile or uncontrolled laughter, fear, apprehension (mild anxiety), crying or absolute terror or anger (frowning), rage or fully depressed or blank and vacant gaze?
- Posture:
    - Was the patient normally relaxed, stiff or guarded?
    - Did he adopt strange postures, which they are capable of maintaining for long period of time?
- **Mannerisms:** Repeated small movements of a habitual kind under stress.
    e.g. characteristics way of raising the eye brow, tick like movements particularly in the perioral area, shrugging of shoulders, repeated clearing of throat, repeated blinking.
- Dress:
    - Was the patient dressed with normal neatness?
    - Were the clothes he wore appropriate to the season and the occasion?
- Hygiene:
    - Was the patient clean, was his hair combed, was his finger nails cut?
- Physical features
    - Looks older or younger than his age
    - Under weight
    - Physical deformity

Inference: Patient was cooperative, rapport was established, eye to eye contact was maintained intermittently. Patient used to change his facial expression with the change of subject, sitting upright, seems to be restless. Patient's dress was appropriate to season, personal hygiene was maintained and looks normal according to his age. There was no history of any physical deformity.

B. MOTOR DISTURBANCES (OBSERVATION)

- **Overactivity or Hyperactivity:** This ranges from mild restlessness and inability to sit still or relax up to the ceaseless of some seriously ill patients. e.g. acute manic reactions.

- **Underactivity or motor retardation:** A general slowing down of activity level and bodily functions.
- **Stupor:** When retardation is progressive and severe and the patient may finally reach a stage where he is completely motionless. He is fully conscious, but remains in one position for hours at a time.
- **Sterotype:** It is the constant repetition of any speech or action. It may also occur in the form of writing a given word or phrase repeatedly.
- **Compulsive movements or compulsion:** The patient feels compelled to carry out a certain pattern of Behavior, while knowing fully well that it is absurd and logically unnecessary yet finding on peace until he was completed it.
- **Echopraxia:** It is the pathological repetition by imitation of the movement of another person. The patient may act as the mirror image of his physician an assume his postures and gestures (is a characteristic of catatonic schizophrenia).
- **Echolalia:** Psychopathological repeating of words or phrases of one person by another; tends to be repetitive and persistent. Seen in certain kinds of schizophrenia, particularly the catatonic types.
- **Negativism:** Patient's failure to co-operate without any apparent reason. It consists of refusal or active resistance to carry out even the simplest request i.e. refusal for food and drink, refusal to void or defecate. Sometimes he may even do the opposite of what he is asked for e.g. lowering his hand when asked to raise it. Push the spoon away instead of putting it into his mouth.
- **Automatic obedience:** It appears the negativism in that the patient shows a pathological degree of compliance (evidenced in waxy flexibility). In other words, commands are followed automatically irrespective of their nature.

Inference: Note if the psychomotor activity is increased, decreased or normal.

EVALUATION OF SPEECH

Note here the form of utterances rather than the content. Does the patient speak spontaneously or only in response of questions?
    Is the amount of speech little or excessive?
    Is it high toned or low toned?
    Is the tempo fast or slow?
    Is it relevant/
    Is it coherent?
    Is the reaction time increased or decreased?
    Is the prosody of speech maintained?

Inference: Describe under these headings: relevance, coherence, volume, tone, tempo, reaction time

DISORDER OF THOUGHT

- Disorders of form of thought
- Disorder of content of thought
- Disorder in rate of speech

Disorder of form of Thought

- **Circumstantiality:** Patient includes in his conversation many unnecessary detail and explanation before the goal is finally reached. The details expressed are related but not essential.
- **Tangential thinking:** It is same as circumstantiality except that the goal is never reached.
  Nurse: Tusi hospital kive ponche c?
  Patient:
  Inference: Present/absent
- **Incoherence:** In which no sense can be extracted from his speech.
- **Irrelevant:** When the patient does not answer appropriately to the question.
  Nurse: Chutti Milan ton baad tusi ghar kive jaoge?

Patient:

Inference: present/absent

- **Neologism:** Patient may his invent his language and use new words. "coinage of new words usually by condensing several other words. Each of which has special meaning for the patient. (present in schizophrenia)
- **Word salad:** Isolated, disconnected words mixed up in a hopeless jumble.
- **Preservation:** Is the involuntary and morbid repetition of a specific word or idea which persists in spite of patients effort to move on to a new idea.

OR

It is persistent response to a prior stimulus after a new stimulus has been presented often with cognitive disorders.

- **Ambivalence or ambivalent ideas:** When two contradictory ideas, emotions, attitudes or wishes exist in the mind of the patient and they are allowed to exist without the rejection of either. It implies dual attitude to a person or object (the attitude being of opposite character).

    Nurse: Ki tuhade family members tuhanu pyar karde ne?

    Patient:

    Inference: Present/absent

Disorders in the Content of Thought (Questioning and Observation)

- **Delusions:** These are false fixed beliefs, which are irrational not shared by persons of same race, age and standard of education, which is held by conviction and which cannot be altered by arguments and which are persistent.

    Systematic delusion: When delusion is built up into complex, elaborate and more fixed structure.

    Unsystematized delusion: When they are fleeting and vague.

There are various type of delusions:

- **Persecutory delusion:** Delusional beliefs of an individual that he is being deliberately interfered with discriminated against, threatened or otherwise mistreated.

    Nurse: Ki tuhanu lagda hai koi tuhanu maarna chaunda hai?

    Patient:

    Inference: Present/absent

- **Delusion of reference:** Delusional beliefs that either people are talking about him referring to him or that the remarks or actions of people he meets are intended to have some special significance for him.

    Nurse: Ki tuhanu lgda k lok sirf tuhade vaare hi gallan karde ne?

    Patient:

    Inference: Present/absent

- **Delusions of influence or passivity:** Delusional beliefs of an individual that enemy is influencing him in many ways and other controls his body, his thoughts and his feelings.

    Nurse: Ki tuhanu lagda hai k koi tuhade vichaar control karda hai?

    Patient:

    Inference: Present/absent

- **Delusions of sin and guilt:** Delusional beliefs of an individual that he has committed some unforgivable sins or committed some wickedness in his past life.

    Nurse: Ki tuhanu lagda hai k eh sab tuhade pichle kite hoye karma da fal hai?

    Patient:

    Inference: Present/absent

- **Hypochondrial delusions:** (Delusions of bodily diseases) are those delusions in which patient hold a fixed conviction concerning the presence of disease or abnormality in some part of his own body.

    Nurse: Ki tuhanu lagda hai k tuhanu koi bimari ho gyi e ya tuhade koi part kharb ho chukka hai?

    Patient:

    Inference: Present/absent

- **Delusions of grandeur:** Delusional beliefs of great power, wealth and influence.

Nurse: Ki tuhade kol koi alag shakti hai jis naal tuc sari duniya nu control kar sakde oo?
Patient:
Inference: Present/absent

- **Delusion of Infidelity (Jealousy):** It is a false belief derived from pathological jealousy that one's lover is unfaithful.
Nurse: Ki tuhanu lagda hai k tuhadi wife da kise naal affair hai?
Patient:
Inference: Present/absent

- **Nihilistic delusion:** Delusional beliefs that nothing exists, that the whole world is destroyed or may be convinced that some fate has been fallen on one or more of his relatives. He may also state that he is dead or that certain part of his body has died or ceased to function. It has two forms:

Depersonalization: When all the things in the environment are changed or destroyed.
Derealisation: When patient says that he himself is changed or dead.
Obsessions: These are persistent, recurrent, intrusive idea, thought or impulse, images that cannot be eliminated from consciousness by logic reasoning. Obsessions are involuntary and ego dystonic.
Nurse: Kde koi kyaal vaar-2 tuhande mann ch aunde ne jo k tuhadi routine nu disturb kar dinde ne te tuahde lyi ohna nu control karna mushkil hunda hai.
Patient:
Inference: Present/absent
Phobia: Persistent, pathological, unrealistic, intense fear of an object or situation.
Nurse: Ki tuhanu kise khass object ton dar lagda?
Patient:
Inference:
Preoccupation: Centering of thought content on a particular idea, associated with a strong affective tone, such as a paranoid trend or a suicidal or homicidal preoccupation.
Nurse: Ki koi khayaal tuhade mann ch vaar aunda?
Patient:
Inference: Present/absent
Phantasy or fantasy: A product of imagination. It is a mental representation of scene or occurrence that is recognized as unreal but is either expected or hoped for.
There are two type of fantasy
- Creative – which prepares for later action.
- Day dreaming – which is the refuge for wishes that cannot be fulfilled in reality.

Disorder of Rate of Speech (Observation)

- **Pressure of speech:** When the rate is accelerated. The speech is valuable that it is difficult for the listener to interrupt (it may also be pressure of flight of ideas). Seen in states of excitement and over activity.
- **Flight of ideas:** When the pressure of talk is more severe there is the tendency of the patient to start talking on one subject and then switch to another then to another with little connection between them.
- **Retardation:** Slowing of speech.
- **Mutism:** The patient may not talk at all (patient may be prevented from speaking by feelings of marked anxiety, fear or hostility).
- **Aphonia:** Patient is able to speak only in a whisper (neurotic patients use the mechanism of conversation).
- **Thought block:** The patient's thought and speech are proceeding at any essentially average rate but are very suddenly and completely interrupted in the middle of sentence, the gap may last for several seconds, even up to a minute after which the patient resumes speaking either where he left off or on a completely new topic.
- **Clang association:** Is an associative disturbance in which the patient may follow one word with another and where the mere sound of a word rather its meaning touches a new thought (there is superficial resemblance of words) e.g. one patient said my life is going with bang, bang, hang, you will hang if you don't watch out.
Inference: Present/absent

DISORDERS OF PERCEPTION (QUESTIONING AND OBSERVATION)

- **Perception:** An act or process of awareness resulting from the act of stimulus upon the sense organs and an additional element coming from the past experiences of the individual.
- **Illusion:** It is defined as subjective perversion of an objective content i.e. the subject himself puts wrong meaning to the subject.
- **Hallucination:** It may be defined as a sensory experience in the absence of a stimulus or an object
- **Auditory hallucinations:** Involving the sense of hearing e.g. the patient may hear voices telling him what to do, communicating on or criticizing his actions. The voices may make accusations, give commands, utter obscene words and suggestions, threaten punishments or provide assurance.
- **Visual hallucinations:** The patient sees vision, usually of clearly defined people or objects, but occasionally flashes of light or representations of geometric patterns and accompanying emotions of joy or terror.
- **Olfactory hallucinations:** Involving the sense of smell. The smell of rarely pleasant one, much more commonly, it is said to be horrible.
- **Gustatory hallucinations:** Involving the sense of taste. It is not complained of as such instead the patent states that his food has a Peculiar smell. Olfactory and gustatory are often found together in one patient.
- **Tactile:** Involving the sense of touch e.g. crawling of ants on the body.
- **Hypnagogic hallucination:** False sensory perception occurring mid between falling sleep and being awake.
- **Hypnopompic hallucination:** False sensory perception occurring midway between sleep awakening.
- **Lilliputian hallucination:** Perception of objects reduced in size.
- **Kinaesthetic hallucination:** False perception of movement or sensation as from and amputated limb (Phantom Limb).
- **Macropsia:** State in which objects appear lager than they are.
- **Micropsia:** State in which objects appear smaller than they are.
- **Mood:** Mood is defined as a pervasive and sustained emotion that colors the person's perception of the world. The psychiatrist is interested in whether the patient remarks voluntarily about feelings or whether it is necessary to ask the patient how he or she feels.
- **Affect:** Affect can be defined as the patient's present emotional responsiveness, inferred from the patient's facial expression, including the amount and the range of expressive Behavior. Affect may or may not be congruent with mood.

Note: When patient is describing his mood observe his facial expression whether these are in accordance with patient's mood.
Inference: is it appropriate to mood or not?

COGNITIVE FUNCTIONS

Insight: Test the patient's level of awareness of his illness,
- Does he think that he is not ill at all ?(absence of insight),
- Does he recognize the presence of illness but gives explanation in physical terms? (Partial insight)
- Does he fully realize the emotional nature of his illness and the cause of his symptoms? (Insight presented)

CLINICAL ASSESSMENT OF COGNITIVE FUNCTIONS

It includes the areas of-
- Orientation
- Attention and concentration
- Memory
- Intelligence
- Judgement

Orientation: Three aspects are described to time, place and person the following questions may be asked in the relevant areas.

Time

- ☐ Approximately what time of the day is it? (if the patient is unable to reply a more specific question may be asked)
- ☐ Is it morning, afternoon, evening or night? (in addition further question may be done to assess estimation of time)
- ☐ Approximately how long id it since you had your breakfast/lunch/tea/dinner? Or approximately how long have I been talking to you?
- ☐ What is the day today? (day of week)
- ☐ What is the date? (day of the month, month , year) today?

Place

- ☐ What place is this? (if the answer is not forthcoming, a specific question is asked)
- ☐ Is this a school, office, hospital, restaurant etc? (if the patient says it is a hospital details may be asked depending in background)

Person

- ☐ Orientation to self is tested by asking the identity of the patient.
- ☐ Inquiring about the identity of the patient's relative or family members.

ATTENTION AND CONCENTRATION

Test used in clinical situation include-
- ☐ The digit span test
- ☐ Serial subtraction
- ☐ Days or months forward to backward

The Digit Span Test

- ☐ **Forward:**
  Patient is given the following instructions- I will be saying some digits , listen to me carefully when I finish saying them, you will have to repeat them in the same order.
    - Gives an example (for example if say 3,7 you say 3,7)
    - Reads digits at the rate of one per second to the patient
    - Notes whether the immediate response of the patient is correct or incorrect. The following digits may be usesd-

5-7-3	4-1-7
5-3-8-	6-1-5-8
1-6-4-9-5	2-9-7-6-3
3-4-1-7-9-6	6-1-5-8-3-9
7-2-5-9-4-8-3	4-7-1-5-3-8-6
4-7-2-9-1-6-8-5	9-2-5-8-3-1-7-4

  The digit span is the highest number of digit repeated correctly.
  The same digits should not be presented more than once – if the patient cannot repeat a particular number of digits on one trial, a trail with the same number of digits is given and credit is given if the response is correct.

- ☐ **Backward:**
  The patient is instructed as follows; I will be saying some digits , listen to me carefully and repeat them after me in a reversed order , for example if I say 2-5 you have to say 5-2. The procedure is the same as for digits forward:
    - The same digits be repeated not be used as for the forward test.
    - No digit backward score is the highest number of digits correctly recalled backward after maximum of 2 trials.

SERIAL SUBTRACTIONS

Increasingly difficult tests are presented. The examiner -
- ☐ Instructs the patient
- ☐ Gives an example of how to perform task
- ☐ Notes the response verbatism and
- ☐ Note the time taken in seconds

Task: Correct response and the limit-
- ☐ 20-1 20 to 0 reversed in 15 secs
- ☐ 40-3 40, 37, 34, 31 etc in 60 secs
- ☐ 100-7 100, 93, 86, 79 etc in 120 secs

Days and months may be asked for in backward to the patient who is familiar with the correct order,

MEMORY

Assessment includes immediate, recent and remote memory
- ☐ Immediate memory- tested by digit span test
- ☐ Recent memory- tested by-
- ☐ **Addressed test-**
  An address consisting of about 4-5 facts which is not known to the patient is slowly read to the patient after instructing him to attend to the examiner. He is engaged in conversation (to avoid rehearsal) and the response is noted verbatism.
- ☐ **Recall** is asked for after 3-5 minutes
  - Asking the patient to recall events in the last 24 hours e.g. details of the time and amount in a meal, visitors to the hospital from an inpatient. Response given by the patient should be noted and cross checked from reliable source.
- ☐ **Remote memory**-information on life events
  - Date of birth or age
  - Numbers of children
  - Names and numbers of family members
  - Time since marriage or death or any family members
  - Year of completing education

4–5 facts may be asked for relevant to the patient background and answer should be cross checked.

INTELLIGENCE

This includes the areas of general information, comprehension, arithmetic and vocabulary.
General information- information relevant to the patient's literacy, age or occupation may be asked e.g. in literature
- ☐ Names of prime minister
- ☐ 5 rivers , cities and states
- ☐ Capitals of countries
- ☐ Current events (major)

For Illiterate

- ☐ Seasons
- ☐ Crops of fruit growing particular season
- ☐ Prices of food grains or food items
- ☐ Prices of land

Comprehension

The ability to understand is questions asked during an interview is index. Specifically the following questions of increasing difficulty may be asked.
- What will you do when you feel cold?
- What will you do if it rains when you start to work?
- What will you do when you miss the bus when you are on a journey?
- What will you do when you find on your that us will be late by the time you ready your work spot?
- Why should we be away from bad company?

Arithmetic

The following questions may be asked with increasing time units.
- How much is 4 rupees and 5 rupees?
- I borrowed 6 rupees from a friend and returned 2 rupees, how much do I still owe to him?
- If a man buys cloth for 12 rupees and gives a shopkeeper 20 rupees, how much change would he get back?
- How many pencils can you buy for 2 rupees of one pencil quarter of a rupees for 25 paise?
- If 18 boys are divide into groups of 6, how many groups will there be?

Time Limits

- 1–3 15 secs
- 4–5 30 secs

Correct answer: 1) 9, 2) 4, 3) 9, 4) 8, 5) 3

Abstraction: Tested by similarities, differences and proverbs.

Similarities: The patient is given the following instructions

I will be giving you some pair of words. You have to tell me in what way they are alike. What is common between them, what is the similarity between them.
- Orange–banana (fruit)
- Dog–lion (animal)
- Eye–ear (sense organs)
- North–west (direction)
- Table–chair (items of furniture)

Note: Correct responses i.e. abstract responses are given in brackets.

Differences: The instructions are as follow

I will be presenting to you some arts of words. Listen carefully and tell me in what they are different from each other.
- **Stone–potato (not edible – edible/ hard – soft)**
- **Fly–butterfly (small – large / nit colorful – colorful)**
- **Cinema–radio (audio– visual audio)**
- **Iron–silver (heavy– light–dull– bright)**
- **Praise–punishment (positive – negative / pleasant – unpleasant)**

PROVERBS

The patient is asked the following questions:
- Whether he knows what a proverb is
- An example of a proverb and what it means

If it is clear that the patient has the concept of a proverb, the following may be asked:
- Slow and steady wins the race

- A barking dogs never bites
- As you sow so shall you reap
- All that glitters is not gold or all that is white is not milk
- Where there is will there is a way
- Empty vessels make more noise
- Every potter praises his pot
- It is useless to cry over split milk

The response of the patient is to be noted verbatism and judged to be correct/incorrect.

Judgement–is assessed in the following areas-
- Personal
- Social
- Test
    - Personal judgement-is assessed by inquiries about the patient future plans
    - Social judgement-is assessed by observation in social situations
    - Test judgement-the following 2 problems are presented to the patient in a manner in which he can be comprehend.
    - Fire problem-If the house in which you are catches fire, what is the first thing you will do (correct answer-try to put off with water)
    - Letter problem-if when you are walking on the roadside you see a stamped and sealed envelope with an address on it which someone had dropped, what will you do?
    (correct answer post it in a letter box or give it to the post man)

General Reaction and Posture

- Attitude voluntary or passive
- Voluntary postures comfortable, natural, constrained or awkward
- What does the patient do if placed in awkward of uncomfortable positions
- Behavior toward physician and nurses; resistive, evasive, irritable, apathetic, complaint.
- Spontaneous acts; any occasional show of playfulness, mischievousness or assaultiveness. Defence movements when interfered with or when pricked with pin, eating and dressing, attention to bowel and bladder. Do the movements show only initial retardation or are they consistent throughout?
- To what extent does the attitude change? If the Behavior occurrence influence the condition?

Practical Record Book of Psychiatric Nursing

FORMAT OF MENTAL STATUS EXAMINATION

Format 1

BIODATA

Name: _____ Age: _____
Sex: _____ Address: _____
Education: _____ Occupation: _____
Marital status: _____ Religion: _____
Socioeconomic status: _____ Informant: _____
Reliability of informant: _____

A. GENERAL APPEARANCE (BY OBSERVATION)

☐ Is the patient co-operative?
_____

☐ Establishment of adequate rapport
_____

☐ Eye contact
_____

☐ Facial expression
_____
_____

☐ Posture
_____

☐ Mannerism
_____

☐ Dress
_____

☐ Hygiene
_____

☐ Physical features
_____
_____

Inference
_____
_____

MOTOR DISTURBANCES (BY OBSERVATION)

☐ Is overactivity or hyperactivity present?
___

☐ Is underactivity or motor retardation present?
___

☐ Is stupor present?
___

☐ Is patient stereotype?
___

☐ Are compulsive movement present?
___

☐ Is echopraxia present?
___

☐ Is echolalia present?
___

☐ Is negativism present?
___

☐ Is automatic obedience present?
___

Inference
___
___
___
___
___

EVALUATION OF SPEECH

Inference
___
___
___
___
___

DISORDER OF THOUGHT

Disorder of form of Thought

Question 1

Answer

Inference

- ☐ Is incoherence present?

- ☐ Is talk irrelevant?

- ☐ Is neologism present?

- ☐ Is word salad present?

- ☐ Is preservation present?

- ☐ Is ambivalence present?

Question 2

Answer

Inference

Disorders in the Content of Thought

Delusions

Persecutory Delusion

Question 1

Answer

Inference

Delusion of Reference

Question 1

Answer

Inference

Delusion of Influence or Passivity

Question 1

Answer

Inference

Delusions of Sin and Guilt

Question 1

Answer

Inference

Hypochondrial Delusions

Question 1

Answer

Inference

Delusions of Grandeur

Question 1

Answer

Inference

Delusion of Infidelity

Question 1

Answer

Inference

Obsessions

Question 1

Answer

Inference

Phobia

Question 1

Answer

Inference

Preoccupation

Question 1

Answer

Inference

Disorder of Rate of Speech (By Observation)

- What is pressure of speech?   Increased/Decreased
- Flights of ideas: Present/Absent
- Is speech retarded?   Yes/No
- Mutism: Present/Absent
- Aphonia: Present/Absent
- Thought block: Present/Absent
- Clang association: Present/Absent

DISORDERS OF PERCEPTION

Illusion

Question 1

Answer

Inference

Hallucinations

Question 1

Answer

Question 2

Answer

Question 3

Answer

Question 4

Answer

Question 5

Answer

Question 6

Answer

Inference

MOOD AND AFFECT

Question 1

Answer

Inference

COGNITIVE FUNCTIONS

Insight

Absent/Partially present/Present

Orientation

Time

Question 1

Answer

Question 2

Answer

Question 3

Answer

Question 4

Answer

Inference

Place

Question 1

Answer

Inference

Person

Question 1

Answer

Inference

Attention and Concentration

Digit Span Test

___

Inference

___

Serial Subtractions

___

Inference

___

Days or Months Forward to Backward

___

Inference

___

Memory

Recent Memory

Question 1

Answer

Inference

Immediate Memory

Question 1

Answer

Inference

Remote Memory

Question 1

Answer

Inference

Intelligence

Question 1

Answer

Question 2

Answer

Question 3

Answer

Inference

Intelligence Test for Illiterate

Question 1

Answer

Question 2

Answer

Question 3

Answer

Inference

Comprehension

Question 1

Answer

Question 2

Answer

Question 3

Answer

Inference

Arithmetic

Question 1

Answer

Question 2

Answer

Question 3

Answer

Inference

Similarities

Question 1

Answer

Question 2

Answer

Question 3

Answer

Inference

Differences

Question 1

Answer

Question 2

Answer

Question 3

Answer

Inference

Proverbs

Question 1

Answer

Question 2

Answer

Question 3

Answer

Inference

Judgement

Fire Test

Question 1

Answer

Inference

Letter Test

Question 1

Answer

Inference

INFERENCE OF MENTAL STATUS EXAMINATION

Practical Record Book of Psychiatric Nursing

FORMAT OF MENTAL STATUS EXAMINATION

Format 2

BIODATA

Name: _____   Age: _____
Sex: _____   Address: _____
Education: _____   Occupation: _____
Marital status: _____   Religion: _____
Socioeconomic status: _____   Informant: _____
Reliability of informant: _____

A. GENERAL APPEARANCE (BY OBSERVATION)

☐ Is the patient co-operative?
_____

☐ Establishment of adequate rapport
_____

☐ Eye contact
_____

☐ Facial expression
_____
_____

☐ Posture
_____

☐ Mannerism
_____

☐ Dress
_____

☐ Hygiene
_____

☐ Physical features
_____
_____

Inference
_____
_____

MOTOR DISTURBANCES (BY OBSERVATION)

☐ Is overactivity or hyperactivity present?

☐ Is underactivity or motor retardation present?

☐ Is stupor present?

☐ Is patient stereotype?

☐ Are compulsive movement present?

☐ Is echopraxia present?

☐ Is echolalia present?

☐ Is negativism present?

☐ Is automatic obedience present?

Inference

EVALUATION OF SPEECH

Inference

DISORDER OF THOUGHT

Disorder of form of Thought

Question 1

Answer

Inference

- ☐ Is incoherence present?

- ☐ Is talk irrelevant?

- ☐ Is neologism present?

- ☐ Is word salad present?

- ☐ Is preservation present?

- ☐ Is ambivalence present?

Question 2

Answer

Inference

Disorders in the Content of Thought

Delusions

Persecutory Delusion

Question 1

Answer

Inference

Delusion of Reference

Question 1

Answer

Inference

Delusion of Influence or Passivity

Question 1

Answer

Inference

Delusions of Sin and Guilt

Question 1

Answer

Inference

Hypochondrial Delusions

Question 1

Answer

Inference

Delusions of Grandeur
Question 1

Answer

Inference

Delusion of Infidelity
Question 1

Answer

Inference

Obsessions
Question 1

Answer

Inference

Phobia
Question 1

Answer

Inference

Preoccupation

Question 1

Answer

Inference

Disorder of Rate of Speech (By Observation)

- What is pressure of speech?   Increased/Decreased
- Flights of ideas: Present/Absent
- Is speech retarded?   Yes/No
- Mutism: Present/Absent
- Aphonia: Present/Absent
- Thought block: Present/Absent
- Clang association: Present/Absent

DISORDERS OF PERCEPTION

Illusion

Question 1

Answer

Inference

Hallucinations

Question 1

Answer

Question 2

Answer

Question 3

Answer

Question 4

Answer

Question 5

Answer

Question 6

Answer

Inference

MOOD AND AFFECT

Question 1

Answer

Inference

COGNITIVE FUNCTIONS

Insight

Absent/Partially present/Present

Orientation

Time

Question 1

Answer

Question 2

Answer

Question 3

Answer

Question 4

Answer

Inference

Place

Question 1

Answer

Inference

Person

Question 1

Answer

Inference

Attention and Concentration

Digit Span Test

_____
_____
_____
_____

Inference
_____

Serial Subtractions

_____
_____
_____
_____

Inference
_____

Days or Months Forward to Backward

_____
_____
_____
_____

Inference
_____

Memory

Recent Memory

Question 1

Answer
_____

Inference

Immediate Memory

Question 1

Answer

Inference

Remote Memory

Question 1

Answer

Inference

Intelligence

Question 1

Answer

Question 2

Answer

Question 3

Answer

Inference

Intelligence Test for Illiterate

Question 1

Answer

Question 2

Answer

Question 3

Answer

Inference

Comprehension

Question 1

Answer

Question 2

Answer

Question 3

Answer

Inference

Arithmetic

Question 1

Answer

Question 2

Answer

Question 3

Answer

Inference

Similarities

Question 1

Answer

Question 2

Answer

Question 3

Answer

Inference

Differences

Question 1

Answer

Question 2

Answer

Question 3

Answer

Inference

Proverbs

Question 1

Answer

Question 2

Answer

Question 3

Answer

Inference

Judgement

Fire Test

Question 1

Answer

Inference

Letter Test

Question 1

Answer

Inference

INFERENCE OF MENTAL STATUS EXAMINATION

Practical Record Book of Psychiatric Nursing

FORMAT OF MENTAL STATUS EXAMINATION

Format 3

BIODATA

Name: _____   Age: _____
Sex: _____   Address: _____
Education: _____   Occupation: _____
Marital status: _____   Religion: _____
Socioeconomic status: _____   Informant: _____
Reliability of informant: _____

A. GENERAL APPEARANCE (BY OBSERVATION)

☐ Is the patient co-operative?
_____

☐ Establishment of adequate rapport
_____

☐ Eye contact
_____

☐ Facial expression
_____
_____
_____

☐ Posture
_____

☐ Mannerism
_____

☐ Dress
_____

☐ Hygiene
_____

☐ Physical features
_____
_____

Inference
_____
_____
_____

MOTOR DISTURBANCES (BY OBSERVATION)

- ☐ Is overactivity or hyperactivity present?

- ☐ Is underactivity or motor retardation present?

- ☐ Is stupor present?

- ☐ Is patient stereotype?

- ☐ Are compulsive movement present?

- ☐ Is echopraxia present?

- ☐ Is echolalia present?

- ☐ Is negativism present?

- ☐ Is automatic obedience present?

Inference

EVALUATION OF SPEECH

Inference

DISORDER OF THOUGHT

Disorder of form of Thought

Question 1

Answer

Inference

☐ Is incoherence present?

☐ Is talk irrelevant?

☐ Is neologism present?

☐ Is word salad present?

☐ Is preservation present?

☐ Is ambivalence present?

Question 2

Answer

Inference

Disorders in the Content of Thought

Delusions

Persecutory Delusion

Question 1

Answer

Inference

Delusion of Reference

Question 1

Answer

Inference

Delusion of Influence or Passivity

Question 1

Answer

Inference

Delusions of Sin and Guilt

Question 1

Answer

Inference

Hypochondrial Delusions

Question 1

Answer

Inference

Delusions of Grandeur

Question 1

Answer

Inference

Delusion of Infidelity

Question 1

Answer

Inference

Obsessions

Question 1

Answer

Inference

Phobia

Question 1

Answer

Inference

Preoccupation

Question 1

Answer

Inference

Disorder of Rate of Speech (By Observation)

- What is pressure of speech?   Increased/Decreased
- Flights of ideas: Present/Absent
- Is speech retarded?   Yes/No
- Mutism: Present/Absent
- Aphonia: Present/Absent
- Thought block: Present/Absent
- Clang association: Present/Absent

DISORDERS OF PERCEPTION

Illusion

Question 1

Answer

Inference

Hallucinations

Question 1

Answer

Question 2

Answer

Question 3

Answer

Question 4

Answer

Question 5

Answer

Question 6

Answer

Inference

MOOD AND AFFECT

Question 1

Answer

Inference

COGNITIVE FUNCTIONS

Insight

Absent/Partially present/Present

Orientation

Time

Question 1

Answer

Question 2

Answer

Question 3

Answer

Question 4

Answer

Inference

Place

Question 1

Answer

Inference

Person

Question 1

Answer

Inference

Attention and Concentration

Digit Span Test

_____
_____
_____
_____
_____

Inference
_____

Serial Subtractions

_____
_____
_____
_____
_____

Inference
_____

Days or Months Forward to Backward

_____
_____
_____
_____
_____

Inference
_____

Memory

Recent Memory

Question 1
_____

Answer
_____

Inference

Immediate Memory

Question 1

Answer

Inference

Remote Memory

Question 1

Answer

Inference

Intelligence

Question 1

Answer

Question 2

Answer

Question 3

Answer

Inference

Intelligence Test for Illiterate

Question 1

Answer

Question 2

Answer

Question 3

Answer

Inference

Comprehension

Question 1

Answer

Question 2

Answer

Question 3

Answer

Inference

Arithmetic

Question 1

Answer

Question 2

Answer

Question 3

Answer

Inference

Similarities

Question 1

Answer

Question 2

Answer

Question 3

Answer

Inference

Differences

Question 1

Answer

Question 2

Answer

Question 3

Answer

Inference

Proverbs

Question 1

Answer

Question 2

Answer

Question 3

Answer

Inference

Judgement

Fire Test

Question 1

Answer

Inference

Letter Test

Question 1

Answer

Inference

INFERENCE OF MENTAL STATUS EXAMINATION

EXAMPLE OF MINI MENTAL STATUS EXAMINATION

Patient's Name: Ram Sarup   Maximum Score: 30   Patient's Score: 24

Component description	Patient score	Points
1. Orientation Ye kon sa saal hai? Kon sa mousam hai? Aaj kon si tarikh hai? Aaj kon sa din hai? Acha abhi kon sa mahena chal rha hai?" "Abhi aap kahan ho. Kon se rajya mein ho? Ye kon sa desh hai? Ye kon sa shehar hai? Ye kon sa hospital hai? Kon si manjil pe abhi aap ho?	1 1 0 0 0 0 0 1 1 1	1 1 1 1 1 1 1 1 1 1
2. Attention and Calculation "kya aap 100 se piche ki taraf paanch aank tak ginti kroge? "Mein aapko ek word dungi aapko uski spelling ulti tarf se bolni hai WORLD backwards." (D-L-R-O-W)	2	5
3. Registration "Mein aapko three word dungi aap unko mere baad dohrana hai?" Orange, apple, banana	3	3
4. Recall "Abhi thodhi der phle mein ne jo teen word btaaye the kya abhi aap unko phir se bologe. Kya aap bta skte ho ki vo kon se teen word the?"	2	3
5. Language 1. "Kya aap bta skte ho ki meinne apne haath mein abhi kya liya hai?" 2. "Kya aap bta skte ho ki meri klaayi pe kya bdha hai?"	1 1	1 1
• "Es line ko dohrana: No ifs, ands, or buts."	0	1
• Mein aapko ek khali kagaj ka tukdha de rahi hun, jo mein bolungi vo aap krna- "Paper ko apne dayein hath mein lo, ab esko aadha fold kro, or esko zamin par rakh do."	3	3
• "Kya aap esko padhoge or jo esmein likha hai vo aap kro." (Written instruction is "Apni ankhein band kro.")	1	1
• "Kya aap apni marzi se koyi bhi line likhoge?" (jis line mein koyi sangya ho.)	1	1
• "Please read this and do what it says." (Written instruction is "Close your eyes.")	1	1
• Mein aapko ek khali kagaj ka tukdha de rahi hun, jo mein bolungi vo aap ko krna hai. • Go through and "Please copy this picture."	1	1
Total Score	24	30

Scoring Key

21–24 as mild cognitive impairment
10–20 as moderate cognitive impairment
<10 as severe cognitive impairment

Conclusion of Mini Mental Status Examination

(Patient is having mild cognitive impairment)

Practical Record Book of Psychiatric Nursing

FORMAT OF MINI MENTAL STATUS EXAMINATION

Format 1

BIODATA

Name: _____   Age: _____
Sex: _____   Address: _____
Education: _____   Occupation: _____
Marital status: _____   Religion: _____
Socioeconomic status: _____   Informant: _____
Reliability of informant: _____

Component description	Patient score	Points
1. Orientation What is the Year? Season? Date? Day of the week? Month?" "Where are we now: State? Country? Town/city? Hospital? Floor?"		
2. Attention and calculation "I would like you to count backward from 100 by sevens." (93, 86, 79, 72, 65, …) Stop after five answers. Alternative: "Spell WORLD backwards." (D-L-R-O-W)		
3. Registration "Can you repeat the name of the 3 objects that I am going to spell right now?" Orange, apple, bnanana		
4. Recall "Earlier I told you the names of three things. Can you tell me what those were?"		

5. Language
  1. "Can you recognize the object that i am holding in my hand?"
  2. "Now recognize the object that I have tied on my wrist?"		

• "Repeat the phrase: 'No ifs, and, or buts."		
• I am giving you a piece of blank paper please follow some instructions— • "Take the paper in your right hand, fold it in half, and put it on the floor."		
• "Please read this and do what it says." (Written instruction is "Close your eyes.")		
• "Make up and write a sentence about anything." (This sentence must contain a noun and a verb)		
• "Please read this and do what it says." (Written instruction is "Close your eyes.")		
• I am giving you a piece of paper having an object drawn by me • Go through and "Please copy this picture."		
Total Score		

Result

Inference

Practical Record Book of Psychiatric Nursing

FORMAT OF MINI MENTAL STATUS EXAMINATION

Format 2

BIODATA

Name: _____ Age: _____
Sex: _____ Address: _____
Education: _____ Occupation: _____
Marital status: _____ Religion: _____
Socioeconomic status: _____ Informant: _____
Reliability of informant: _____

Component description	Patient score	Points
1. Orientation What is the Year? Season? Date? Day of the week? Month?" "Where are we now: State? Country? Town/city? Hospital? Floor?"		
2. Attention and calculation "I would like you to count backward from 100 by sevens." (93, 86, 79, 72, 65, …) Stop after five answers. Alternative: "Spell WORLD backwards." (D-L-R-O-W)		
3. Registration "Can you repeat the name of the 3 objects that I am going to spell right now?" Orange, apple, bnanana		
4. Recall "Earlier I told you the names of three things. Can you tell me what those were?"		

5. Language
  1. "Can you recognize the object that i am holding in my hand?"
  2. "Now recognize the object that I have tied on my wrist?"		

• "Repeat the phrase: 'No ifs, and, or buts."		
• I am giving you a piece of blank paper please follow some instructions— • "Take the paper in your right hand, fold it in half, and put it on the floor."		
• "Please read this and do what it says." (Written instruction is "Close your eyes.")		
• "Make up and write a sentence about anything." (This sentence must contain a noun and a verb)		
• "Please read this and do what it says." (Written instruction is "Close your eyes.")		
• I am giving you a piece of paper having an object drawn by me • Go through and "Please copy this picture."		
Total Score		

Result

Inference

Practical Record Book of Psychiatric Nursing

FORMAT OF MINI MENTAL STATUS EXAMINATION

Format 3

BIODATA

Name: _____   Age: _____
Sex: _____   Address: _____
Education: _____   Occupation: _____
Marital status: _____   Religion: _____
Socioeconomic status: _____   Informant: _____
Reliability of informant: _____

Component description	Patient score	Points
1. Orientation What is the Year? Season? Date? Day of the week? Month?" "Where are we now: State? Country? Town/city? Hospital? Floor?"		
2. Attention and calculation "I would like you to count backward from 100 by sevens." (93, 86, 79, 72, 65, …) Stop after five answers. Alternative: "Spell WORLD backwards." (D-L-R-O-W)		
3. Registration "Can you repeat the name of the 3 objects that I am going to spell right now?" Orange, apple, bnanana		
4. Recall "Earlier I told you the names of three things. Can you tell me what those were?"		
5. Language 1. "Can you recognize the object that i am holding in my hand?" 2. "Now recognize the object that I have tied on my wrist?"		
• "Repeat the phrase: 'No ifs, and, or buts.'"		
• I am giving you a piece of blank paper please follow some instructions— • "Take the paper in your right hand, fold it in half, and put it on the floor."		
• "Please read this and do what it says." (Written instruction is "Close your eyes.")		
• "Make up and write a sentence about anything." (This sentence must contain a noun and a verb)		
• "Please read this and do what it says." (Written instruction is "Close your eyes.")		
• I am giving you a piece of paper having an object drawn by me • Go through and "Please copy this picture."		
Total Score		

Result

Inference

EXAMPLE FOR PROCESS RECORDING

DEFINITION

Process recording is a written account or verbatim recording of all that transpired/emerged, during and immediately following the nurse-patient interaction.

In other words, it is the recording of the conversation during the interaction or the interview between the nurse and patient in the psychiatric set up with the nurse's inference. It may be written during the interaction or immediately after the one to one interaction.

PRE-REQUISITE FOR PROCESS RECORDING

Physical Setting

Calm and quiet environment (Interview rooms or bed side, if separate room is not available)
   Obtaining consent from patient for recording the information.
   Maintain confidentiality of information.

Features of Process Recording

- Mention date, time and duration of interaction.
- Record nurses own thoughts and feelings before interaction.
- Reason for choosing the patient for process recording.
- Objectives should be formulated prior to meeting and function as a guide for interaction.
- Record the overall response of patient towards the interaction.
- Record the communication techniques used by nurses.
- Time required to record is 30 min (20 min for active interactions, 10 min for conclusion and planning for next interview).
- The recording process should end with a brief summary to evaluate whether the initial objectives for the interaction were met.

EXAMPLE FOR PROCESS RECORDING

BIODATA

Name: Mr. Kumar

Sex: Male

Bed No.: 18

Education: Graduation

Marital Status: Married

Language: Hindi

Age: 46 years

Ward: Open Male Ward

Address: Kuthala Ghat, Bhopal

Occupation: Self employed

Income: 35000/- PM

Date of Admission: 12/6/2018

PRESENT COMPLAINTS

According to Patient

- Mann udas rehta hai.
- Kuch bhi acha nahi lagta.
- Mar jane ko dil karta hai.

According to Relatives

- Sara din chup rahta hai.
- Kuch nahi khata.
- Kissi se baat nahi karta.
- Kabhi kabhi rone lagta hai
- 2 baar suicide karne kee koshish kee

HISTORY OF PRESENTING COMPLAINTS

From the last 2 months he is showing the above mentioned symptoms. Now he tried to commit suicide.

OBJECTIVES OF INTERVIEW

Patient's point of view (Students may write 2 or 3 objectives. These are the list of possible objectives for reference only)
- To establish rapport and therapeutic IPR
- To socialize effectively
- To ventilate his feelings
- To identify the problems
- To learn healthy coping mechanisms
- To develop health life style
- To learn regarding medications and its importance
- To develop and maintain insight
- To get back pre-morbid personality
- To get prepared for discharge /termination of IPR

Student's point of view: (Students may write 2 or 3 objectives. These are the list of possible objectives for reference only)
- ☐ To develop adequate communication skill
- ☐ To develop confidence in maintaining therapeutic relationship
- ☐ To develop skill in acknowledging the problems of the patient
- ☐ To assist the patient in dealing with his personal problems
- ☐ To assist the patient in developing positive coping mechanisms
- ☐ To procure skill in evaluating the pre-set objectives in order to assess the effectiveness of therapeutic IPR
- ☐ To judge self in dealing with anxiety, fear and sentiments while progressing through the therapeutic IPR

First interview

Date: 17/06/2018 **Time:** 11:30am
Duration: 15-30 min. **Specific objectives:** To establish therapeutic IPR

Participants	Conversation	Therapeutic Communication Technique	Inference
N	Good morning Kumar.	Greeting the patient	Checking social judgment
P	Good morning sister		
N	Mera naam rani hai. Mai ek nursing student hoon. Mai aap se baat karna chahti hoon. Kya app mujh se baatkroge?	Introducing oneself	Checking his willingness to participate in interview
P	Hnji zarur		
N	Aap kaise ho aaj?	Questioning	Starting with non threatening issues to develop rapport Checking memory of the patient
P	Mai theek hoon.		
N	Aap kis din admit hue?	Exploring	Checking orientation of the patient
P	Mein 16sept. ko admit hua tha.		
N	Abhi aap ke saath kaun hai?	Exploring	Checking insight of the patient
P	Abhi mere saath meri mother hai		
N	Aap ees hospital mein kis vajah se admit huye the?	Exploring	Checking social judgment
P	Maine 2-3 suicide attempt karne ki koshish ki thi.		
N	Aisi kya baat huyi thi k aap ne suicide karne ki koshish ki thi.	Giving broad opening	Checking insight of the patient
P	Ye mai aap ko kisi aur din batauga. Abhi mujhe neend a rhi hai.		
N	Cholo theek hai. Thik hai phir kal mein same time pe aap ke saath baat karungi	Giving confirmation	Planning for next interview
P	Hnj imai baat karunga.		

Summary

Kumar was very co-operative thorough out the interview. The objective of this interview was to establish IPR with Kumar. He is willing to continue with the interview.

Evaluation

I was able to establish therapeutic relationship with client

Introspection

- I was able to conduct the interview confidently.
- I did not find any problem during interview.
- I was able to establish therapeutic relationship.

Plan for the next interview

I planned to discuss about family members and his friends in the next interview.

FORMAT OF PROCESS RECORDING

Format 1

BIODATA

Name: _____ Age: _____

Sex: _____ Address: _____

Education: _____ Occupation: _____

Marital status: _____ Religion: _____

Socioeconomic status: _____ Informant: _____

Reliability of informant: _____

PRE-REQUISITE FOR PROCESS RECORDING

_____
_____
_____
_____

DATE, TIME AND DURATION OF INTERACTION

_____
_____
_____

REASON FOR CHOOSING THE PATIENT FOR PROCESS RECORDING

_____
_____
_____
_____

OBJECTIVE/S OF PROCESS RECORDING

_____
_____
_____
_____

PROCESS RECORDING

_____
_____
_____
_____

SUMMARY

_____
_____
_____
_____
_____
_____
_____

PLAN FOR THE NEXT INTERVIEW

FORMAT OF PROCESS RECORDING

Format 2

BIODATA

Name: _____ Age: _____

Sex: _____ Address: _____

Education: _____ Occupation: _____

Marital status: _____ Religion: _____

Socioeconomic status: _____ Informant: _____

Reliability of informant: _____

PRE-REQUISITE FOR PROCESS RECORDING

_____
_____
_____
_____

DATE, TIME AND DURATION OF INTERACTION

_____
_____
_____

REASON FOR CHOOSING THE PATIENT FOR PROCESS RECORDING

_____
_____
_____
_____

OBJECTIVE/S OF PROCESS RECORDING

_____
_____
_____

PROCESS RECORDING

SUMMARY

_____
_____
_____
_____
_____
_____
_____

PLAN FOR THE NEXT INTERVIEW

FORMAT OF PROCESS RECORDING

Format 3

BIODATA

Name: _____ Age: _____

Sex: _____ Address: _____

Education: _____ Occupation: _____

Marital status: _____ Religion: _____

Socioeconomic status: _____ Informant: _____

Reliability of informant: _____

PRE-REQUISITE FOR PROCESS RECORDING

_____
_____
_____
_____

DATE, TIME AND DURATION OF INTERACTION

_____
_____
_____

REASON FOR CHOOSING THE PATIENT FOR PROCESS RECORDING

_____
_____
_____
_____

OBJECTIVE/S OF PROCESS RECORDING

_____
_____
_____

PROCESS RECORDING

SUMMARY

_____
_____
_____
_____
_____
_____
_____

PLAN FOR THE NEXT INTERVIEW

Practical Record Book of Psychiatric Nursing

EXAMPLE OF NURSING CARE PLAN

IDENTIFICATION DATA

Client name	: Mr. Suyog khana	**Age**	: 35 Years
Sex	: Male	**Father**	: Mr. Rajender khana
Address	: Raipura(M.P)	**Education**	: Law.
Occupation	: Lawyer	**Income**	: 35000
Marital status	: Married	**Religion**	: Hindu
Date of admission	: 12/03/2016	**Diagnosis**	: Depression

INFORMANT

Mother and wife and both are reliable.

PRESENTING CHIEF COMPLAINTS

According to Patient

- Restlessness,
- Irritability
- Lack of confidence
- Feelings of discomfort,
- Helplessness
- Decreased ability to communicate verbally
- Repeated thoughts related to particular events
- Worries about future and family members
- Decreased sleep
- Decreased appetite

According to Informant

- Inability to experience pleasure
- Sleep disturbances
- Suicidal behavior
- Not taking food
- Talking to self
- Hypoactive
- Hopelessness
- Helplessness

HISTORY OF PRESENT ILLNESS

Mr. Suyog khana was apparently normal before two years. He lost his father due to Hypertension. Since that time he developed these symptoms. He was not interesting to do work. He was not taking proper food. He was having continuous feeling of hopelessness and insomnia. On 12/03/2016 he was brought in Mental hospital Gwalior under psychiatry department and diagnosed as Depression disorder and admitted in male open ward for further evaluation and treatment.

TREATMENT HISTORY

Mr. Suyog khana did not go for any psychiatric treatment before. At present patient receiving Tab. carbamazepine – 50 mg/day, Tab. Olanzapine – 25 mg/day and Tab. Clonazepam – 1 mg/day along with yoga therapy, individual psychotherapy, group therapy and family counseling.

PAST PSYCHIATRIC HISTORY

No significant data found related to the psychiatric illness in past life.

PAST MEDICAL HISTORY

Mr. Suyog khana did not have any major medical illness history.

PAST SURGICAL HISTORY

There is no significant data found for surgical history.

FAMILY HISTORY

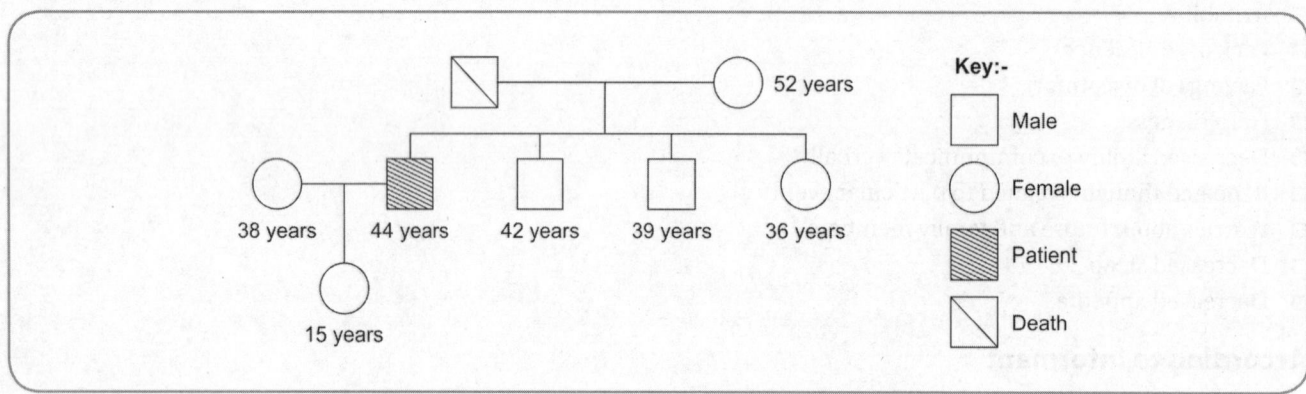

SOCIO-ECONOMIC HISTORY

Mr. suyog khana is a lawyer. He and his brothers are the earning members in his family. His monthly family income is 35000/ per month. He belongs to a middle class family. He is living in ranted house. Electricity and water facility is available in house. Drainage is proper.

PERSONAL HISTORY

Perinatal History

Mr. Suyog khana was delivered at full term by normal vaginal delivery. He cried immediately after birth and there was no postnatal complication like cyanosis, convulsions and jaundice.

Childhood History

Primary caregiver was mother. Weaning started at the age of 11 months and all developmental milestones was achieved at appropriate age period. He was very much emotionally attached with his mother and getting easily emotionally disturbed.

Educational History

Education was started at the age of 3 years. He was average in academic performance and had good relationships with teachers and peers. He never dropout from school. He left the education after finishing his law and started to go for earning.

Play History

He used to play with both sex peer group and had good relationship with peers.

Emotional Problems During Adolescence

In his adolescence period he was very much emotionally attached with his mother and father and got easily emotionally disturbed.

Puberty

Secondary sexual characteristics appeared at the age of 14 years. He did not have anxious mood regarding sexual changes.

Occupational history

Mr. Suyog khana is a lawyer. He was performing well in his work but after death of his father he lost interest in the work. He is having less number of friends.

Premorbid Personality

- ☐ Interpersonal relationships : Introvert
- ☐ Use of leisure time : Watching movies on TV
- ☐ Predominant mood : Easily get irritated, immediate reaction to stressful events
- ☐ Attitude to self and others : Positive and hostile.
- ☐ Attitude to work and responsibility : He was going regular to work and never try to escape from responsibilities for any task.
- ☐ Religious beliefs and moral attitude : Having more faith on religious and participating in religious activity.
- ☐ Fantasy life : No complaint of daydreaming.
- ☐ Habits : He is not having any habit like smoking and drinking.

PHYSICAL EXAMINATION

S. No.	Vital sign	Normal value	Patient's value
1.	Temperature	98.6°F	99.0°F
2.	Pulse	72–90 beats/min	78 beats/min
3.	Respiration	14–20 breath/min	16 breath/min
4.	Blood pressure	120/80 mm of Hg	120/80 mm of Hg

During physical examination all the findings were found normal in head to foot examination and there is no clinically significant finding.

MENTAL STATUS EXAMINATION

General Appearance and Behavior

- Appearance : Looking dull and anxious
- Level of grooming : Poorly Groomed
- Level of cleanliness : Unhygienic
- Level of consciousness : Conscious
- Mode of entry : Persuaded by family
- Cooperativeness : Cooperative
- Eye-to-eye contact : Not Maintained
- Psychomotor activity : Decreased activity
- Rapport : Established properly
- Gesturing : Exaggerated
- Posturing : Closed posture
- Other catatonic phenomena : Not present
- Conversion and dissociative signs : Not present
- Compulsive acts or rituals : Not present
- Hallucinatory behavior : Some time talking to self

Speech

- Student Nurse : What is your name?
- Client : Suyog Khana
- Initiation : Patient responded when talk
- Reaction time : Normal
- Rate : Normal
- Productivity : Elaborate speech
- Volume : Normal
- Tone : Normal tone
- Relevance : Relevant
- Stream : Tangential
- Coherence : Fully associated
- Others : No rhyming, punning, echolalia perseveration.

Mood

- Subjective
  Student nurse : How do you feel?
  Patient : I am anxious about my future and my family.
- Objective : Anxious and furious with confused mood.

Thought

Student nurse : What type of the ideas comes in your mind?
Client : I am not able to think about my future and having worry about my family.

- Stream : Pressure of thoughts.
- Form : Unwanted thought

- **Content**
  Student nurse : Do you feel that someone may harm you?
  Client : Who will harm me! but it is very difficult to live.
  Remarks : Suicidal thought.

Perception

- **Hallucinations**
  Student nurse : Do you hear any sound or see someone whenever you are alone?
  Client : Yes some time my father's voice I can hear.
  Remarks : Auditory hallucinations present

Cognitive Functions

- **Consciousness**
  Student nurse : Hello, Mr. Suyog Khana
  Client : Yes sir
  Remarks : Patient has obeyed by calling his name
- **Orientation**
  - **Person**
  Student nurse : Who is sitting nearby you?
  Client : My Brother and my mother
  Remarks : Oriented to person
  - **Place**
  Student nurse : Where are you now?
  Client : I am in Mental hospital Gwalior
  Remarks : Oriented to place
  - **Time**
  Student nurse : What is the day today?
  Client : Wednesday
  Remarks : Oriented to time
- **Attention**
  Student nurse : Repeat the digit backward 2, 4, 6, 8, 10.
  Client : 10, 8…4..6..2.
  Remarks : Attention aroused with difficulty
- **Concentration**
  Student nurse : Name the months in backward?
  Client : December, November…September, October, June, July … August, March ….January.
  Remarks : Concentration sustained with difficulty
- **Memory**
  - **Immediate**
  Student nurse : Repeat the word what I say Table, Pen, Rose, Bus and Tree.
  Client : Table, Pen, Rose, Bus and Tree
  Remarks : Immediate memory present
  - **Recent**
  Student nurse : What you had in breakfast?
  Client : Parantha with curd
  Remarks : Recent memory present

- **Remote**

  Student nurse : When is your birthday?

  Client : han......................12th June

  Remarks : Remote memory poor

- **Intelligence**

  Student nurse : Who is the Prime Minister of India?

  Client : Narendra Modi

  Remarks : Normal intelligence

- **Abstraction**

  Student nurse : What you will do if you see fire in your neighbor house?

  Client : I will call upon fire brigade.

Insight: (Grade 1 to 6)

Student Nurse : Do you accept your illness and require treatment?

Client : Yes, I am feeling helpless and hearing father's voice.

Remarks : Grade 6 Insight is present

Judgment

Student Nurse : What you will you do if you find "Close latter on the road"?

Client : I should not touch.

Remarks : Judgment is impaired

INVESTIGATION

Sl. No	Investigations	Patient's value	Normal value
1.	Blood		
	• Heamoglobin	13 g/dL	13–15
	• Red blood cell	4.8 mil/cmm	4.5–6.51
	• PCV	38.2%	20–54
	• Platelets	2.89 lacs	1.5–4.5
	• Total WBC different count	9700 cu/mm	5000–11000
	• Lymphocytes	37%	20–45
	• Esinophills	3%	1–6
	• Monocytes	4%	1–6
	• MCV	87 fl	80–99
	• MCH	30 pg	27–33
	• MCHC	33.7 g/dL	32–37
	• ESR	14 mm/hr	0–20
	Routine Investigation		
	• RBS	129 mgs/dL	< 150
	• Blood urea	28 mg/dL	20–45
	• S. creatinine	1.0 mgs/dL	0.7–1.2
	• S. sodium	137 mEq/L	135–145
	• S. potassium	4.4 mEq/L	3.5–4.5
	LFT		
	• S. bilirubin	0.9 mgs/dL	1
	• S. total protein	6.5 gm/dL	6–8
	• S. albumin	4.2 gm/dL	3–5
	• S. globulin	2.2 gm/dL	1.8–3.6
	• Alkaline phosphate	64 IU/L	80–120

MEDICATION CHART

- Tab. Fluoxetine – 50 mg/day,
- Tab. Olanzapine – 25 mg/day and
- Tab. Clonazepam – 1 mg/day

Sl. No.	Trade name	Pharmacological name	Group	Doses	Route	Frequency	Action	Indication	Contra-Indications	Side-effects	Nsg. Responsibility
1.	Prodep	Fluoxetine	SSRI	50 mg	Oral	BD	It block the serotonin reuptake channel and increase serotonin level at post-synaptic space.	Depressive episode, depression with psychotic symptoms, dysthymia, ADHD, panic attack, PTSD and ADS.	Severe renal failure, hypersensitivity, concomitant MAOI's	Constipation, urinary retention, hypotension, impotence, priapism, sedation	• Check the physician's order. • Medication given must be charted on the patient's case sheet. • Check the five rights for drug administration • Always address the patient by name and make certain identification • Do not leave the patient until the drug is swallowed • Do not allow the patient to carry drugs • Do not force oral medication • Check drug daily • Observe for drug specific side-effects • Instruct the family members when to contact psychiatrist
2.	Epitral	Clonazepam	BDZ	1 mg	Oral	BD	It act on BDZ receptor I and II and enhance GABA transmission in the brain.	Generalized anxiety disorder, panic disorder, agoraphobia, sleep disorder, convulsion, alcohol dependence, acute mania and narcoanalysis.	Hypersensitivity, pulmonary insufficiency, respiratory depression	Drowsiness, somnolence, fatigue, vertigo, loss of libido	
3.	Zyprexa	Olanzapine	Anti psychotic	25 mg	Oral	OD	Acts only on the mesolimbic system.	Apathy, decreased sociality, anhedonia, chronic schizophrenia, Acute psychoses, delusional disorders, and hallucinations	Hypersensitivity, MI, hepatic imparimment	Common sedation Hypotension, Diabetes and EPS may and may not be present	

OTHER THERAPEUTIC THERAPIES

- ☐ Yoga therapy
- ☐ Individual psychotherapy
- ☐ Group therapy
- ☐ Family counseling

Assessment Techniques

- ☐ Observation
- ☐ Communication
- ☐ Interview

Summary

Mr. Suyog Khana is a case of depression. He is responding minimum, anxious, having loss of appetite, loss of interest, suicidal gesture, helplessness, worry about family, have auditory hallucination and inferiority feeling. His immediate and recent memory is intact but remote memory is poor and he is not able to take decision.

NURSING PROCESS

Nursing Diagnosis

- ☐ Ineffective coping related to inability to form a valid appraisal of the stressors and inability to use available resources evidenced by suicidal ideas.
- ☐ Disturbed sensory perception auditory related to withdrawal into the self as evidenced by inappropriate responses
- ☐ Anxiety related to environmental conflict evidenced by client focus on self and tendency to become rattled.
- ☐ Impaired social interaction related to insufficient or excessive quantity or ineffective quality of social exchange evidenced by withdrawn behavior.

Practical Record Book of Psychiatric Nursing

Nsg. Diagnosis	Goals	Intervention	Implementation	Evaluation
1. Ineffective coping related to inability to form a valid appraisal of the stressors and inability to use available resources evidenced by suicidal ideas.	Be free from self-inflicted harm evidenced by express feelings directly with congruent verbal and nonverbal messages	• Provide a safe environment for the client. • Continually assess the client's potential for suicide. • Observe the client closely, especially after antidepressant medication begins to raise the client's mood • Reorient the client to person, place, and time as indicated • Spend time with the client. • Initially, assign the same staff members to work with the client whenever possible. • When first communicating with the client, use simple, direct sentences; avoid complex sentences or directions.	• Provided a safe environment for the client. • Continually assessed the client's potential for suicide. • Observed the client closely, especially After antidepressant medication begins to raise the client's mood • Reoriented the client to person, place, and time as indicated • Spent time with the client. • Initially, assigned the same staff members to work with the client whenever possible. • When first communicating with the client, used simple, direct sentences; avoid complex sentences or directions.	Client free from self-inflicted harm evidenced by express feelings directly with congruent verbal and nonverbal messages
2. Disturbed sensory perception (auditory/visual) related to withdrawal into the self as evidenced by inappropriate responses	Maintain the normal sensory perception and eliminate the hallucinations	• Observe the client for sings of hallucinations. • Avoid touching the client without warning. • Do not reinforce the hallucinations. • Distract the client from the hallucinations. • Encourage the client to share hallucinations.	• Observed the client (pt has talking to self) • Maintain the IPR and distance. • Encouraged his self esteem. • Tried to involve in personal tasks.	Client able to define the reality and eliminate the hallucinations in some extent
3. Anxiety related to environmental conflict evidenced by client focus on self and tendency to become rattled	Patient will experience reduced anxiety by identified precipitant situations	• Identify feelings to keep them from interfering with treatment • Accept patient as is • Explore factors that precipitate phobic reactions and anxiety. • Reassure patient he is safe • Support patient with desensitization techniques to help him overcome problem • Give patient chance to ventilate feelings. • Teach relaxation techniques such as breathing exercises, progressive muscles relaxation, guided imagery • Help patient set limits and compromises on behavior where ready and allow patient to be afraid. Fear is a feeling, neither right nor wrong.	• Identified feelings to keep them from interfering with treatment • Accepted patient as is • Explored factors that precipitate phobic reactions and anxiety. • Reassured patient he is safe • Supported patient with desensitization techniques to help him overcome problem. • Given patient chance to ventilate feelings. • Taught relaxation techniques such as breathing exercises, progressive muscles relaxation, guided imagery • Helped patient set limits and compromises on behavior where ready and allow patient to be afraid. Fear is a feeling, neither right nor wrong.	Patient experienced reduced anxiety by identified precipitant situations

Contd...

Nsg. Diagnosis	Goals	Intervention	Implementation	Evaluation
4. Impaired social interaction related to insufficient or excessive quantity or ineffective quality of social exchange evidenced by withdrawn behavior	To improve social interaction evidenced by patient will communicate with others	• Teach the client social skills, and encourage him or her to practice these skills with staff members and other clients. • Initially, interact with the client on a one-to-one basis. Progress to facilitating social interactions between the client and other clients, then in small groups and gradually larger groups. • Encourage the client to pursue personal interests, hobbies, and recreational activities. Consultation with a recreational therapist may be indicated. • Encourage the client to identify supportive people outside the hospital and to develop these relationships.	• Teach the client social skills, and encourage him or her to practice these skills with staff members and other clients. • Initially, interact with the client on a one-to-one basis. Progress to facilitating social interactions between the client and other clients, then in small groups and gradually larger groups. • Encourage the client to pursue personal interests, hobbies, and recreational activities. Consultation with a recreational therapist may be indicated. • Encourage the client to identify supportive people outside the hospital and to develop these relationships.	Improved social interaction evidenced by patient will communicate with others

HEALTH EDUCATION

- Support patient with desensitization techniques to help him overcome problem
- Give patient chance to ventilate feelings.
- Teach relaxation techniques such as breathing exercises, progressive muscles relaxation, guided imagery
- Help patient set limits and compromises on behavior where ready and allow patient to be afraid. Fear is a feeling, neither right nor wrong.
- Health education given regarding nutrition.
- Encourage social interaction.
- Sleep and hygiene techniques.
- Family's to use alternative coping methods.
- Taught about the positive coping methods.
- Prevention of self harm.
- Advised to spend more time with family.
- Avoid conveying to the client the belief that hallucinations are real. Do not converse with the "voices" or otherwise reinforce the client's belief in the hallucinations as reality
- Educated the patient and family members regarding medication- dosage and side effects of the medication.
- Advice the patient for regular checks up and follows up.

Discharge Plan

Patient not yet discharged and receiving treatments.

Summary

Mr. Suyog khana brought to the psychiatric ward on 12/03/16 with the complaints of decreased attention span, restlessness, irritability, lack of confidence, poor impulse control, feelings of discomfort, helplessness, hypoactivity, perceptual field deficits, decreased ability to communicate verbally, repeated thoughts related to particular events, worries about future and family members, decreased sleep, decreased appetite, inability to experience pleasure, sleep disturbances, suicidal behavior, not taking food, and talking to self.

He is diagnosed as a case of depression.

BIBLIOGRAPHY

- Townsend.M, (2007), "Psychiatric Mental Health Nursing", Jaypee brothers, New Delhi, India.
- Doenges M.E. et al., (1995), "Psychiatric Care Plans Guidelines for Planning and Documenting Client Care", 2nd ed. F. A. Davis Company, Philadelphia, PA.
- Ahuja.N, (2006), "A Short Text Book of Psychiatry", Jaypee brothers, New Delhi, India.
- Sreevani.R, (2008), "A Guide to Mental Health and Psychiatric Nursing", Jaypee Brothers, New Delhi, India.

FORMAT OF NURSING CARE PLAN

Format 1

Identification Data

Client name: _____   Age: _____
Sex: _____   Father: _____
Address: _____   Education: _____
Occupation: _____   Income: _____
Marital status: _____   Religion: _____
Date of admission: _____   Diagnosis: _____

Informant

_____
_____
_____
_____

Presenting Chief Complaints

According to Patient

_____
_____
_____
_____

According to Informant

_____
_____
_____
_____

History of Present Illness

_____
_____
_____
_____
_____

Treatment History

Past Psychiatric History

Past Medical History

Past Surgical History

Family History

Genogram

Socio-economic History

Personal History

Prenatal History

Childhood History

Educational History

Play History

Emotional Problems during Adolescence

_____
_____
_____
_____
_____

Puberty

_____
_____
_____
_____

Occupational History

_____
_____
_____
_____
_____

Premorbid Personality

Interpersonal relationships

_____

Use of leisure time

_____

Predominant mood

_____

Attitude to self and others

_____

Attitude to work and responsibility

_____

Religious beliefs and moral attitudes

_____

Fantasy life

_____

Habits

_____

PHYSICAL EXAMINATION

S. No.	Vital sign	Normal value	Patient's value
1.	Temperature	98.6°F	
2.	Pulse	72–90 beats/min	
3.	Respiration	14–20 breath/min	
4.	Blood pressure	120/80 mm Hg	

MENTAL STATUS EXAMINATION

General Appearance and Behavior

Appearance

_____

Level of grooming

_____

Level of cleanliness

_____

Level of consciousness

Mode of entry

Cooperativeness

Eye-to-eye contact

Psychomotor activity

Rapport

Gesturing

Posturing

Other movements

Other catatonic phenomena

Conversion and dissociative signs

Compulsive acts or rituals

Hallucinatory behavior

Inference:

Speech
Student Nurse:

Client
Initiation

Reaction time

Rate

Productivity

___

Volume

___

Tone

___

Relevance

___

Stream

___

Coherence

___

Others

___

Mood

Subjective:

___

Student nurse:

___

<u>Patient</u>:

___

Objective:
Thought

Student Nurse

Client:

Stream

Form

Content

Student nurse:

Client:
Remarks:

Perception

Hallucinations

Student Nurse:

Client:
Remarks:

Cognitive Functions

Consciousness

Student Nurse:

Client:
Remarks

Orientation

Person

Student Nurse:

Client:
Remarks

Student Nurse:

Client:
Remarks

Time

Student Nurse

Client:
Remarks

Attention

Student Nurse:

Client:
Remarks

Concentration

Student Nurse:

Client:
Remarks

Memory

Immediate

Student Nurse:

Client:
Remarks

Recent

Student Nurse:

Client:
Remarks:

_____

_____

Remote

_____

Student Nurse:

_____

Client
Remarks

_____

_____

Intelligence

_____

Student Nurse

_____

Client:
Remarks

_____

_____

Abstraction

_____

Student Nurse:

Client:
Remarks

Insight: (grade1 to 6)

Student Nurse:

Client
Remarks

Judgment

Student Nurse:

Client:
Remarks:

INVESTIGATION

Sl. No	Investigations	Patient's value	Normal value
1.	Blood		
	• Heamoglobin		13–15
	• Red blood cell		4.5–6.51
	• PCV		20–54
	• Platelets		1.5–4.5
	• Total WBC different count		5000–11000
	• Lymphocytes		20–45
	• Eosinophils		1–6
	• Monocytes		1–6
	• MCV		80–99
	• MCH		27–33
	• MCHC		32–37
	• ESR		0–20
	Routine investigation		
	• RBS		<150
	• Blood urea		20–45
	• S. creatinine		0.7–1.2
	• S. sodium		135–145
	• S. potassium		3.5–4.5
	LFT		
	• S. bilirubin		1
	• S. total protein		6–8
	• S. albumin		3–5
	• S. globulin		1.8–3.6
	• Alkaline phosphate		80–120

MEDICATION CHART/DRUG SHEET

Sl. No.	Trade name	Pharmacological name	Group	Doses	Route	Frequency	Action	Indication	Contraindications	Side-effects	Nursing responsibility
1.											
2.											
3.											

Contd...

Practical Record Book of Psychiatric Nursing

Sl. No.	Trade name	Pharmacological name	Group	Doses	Route	Frequency	Action	Indication	Contraindications	Side-effects	Nursing responsibility
4.											
5.											
6.											

228

OTHER THERAPEUTIC THERAPIES

Assessment Techniques

Summary

Nursing Process

Nursing Diagnosis

Practical Record Book of Psychiatric Nursing

Nursing diagnose	Goals	Intervention	Implementation	Evaluation

Contd...

Nursing diagnosis	Goals	Planning	Implementation	Evaluation

Contd...

Nursing diagnosis	Goals	Planning	Implementation	Evaluation

Health Education

Discharge Plan

SUMMARY

BIBLIOGRAPHY

FORMAT OF NURSING CARE PLAN

Format 2

Identification Data

Client name: _____ Age: _____
Sex: _____ Father: _____
Address: _____ Education: _____
Occupation: _____ Income: _____
Marital status: _____ Religion: _____
Date of admission: _____ Diagnosis: _____

Informant

_____
_____
_____
_____

Presenting Chief Complaints

According to Patient

_____
_____
_____
_____

According to Informant

_____
_____
_____
_____

History of Present Illness

_____
_____
_____
_____

Treatment History
_____
_____
_____

Past Psychiatric History
_____
_____
_____
_____

Past Medical History
_____
_____
_____
_____

Past Surgical History
_____
_____
_____

Family History
_____
_____
_____
_____

Genogram
_____
_____
_____

Socio-economic History

Personal History

Prenatal History

Childhood History

Educational History

Play History

Emotional Problems during Adolescence

Puberty

Occupational History

Premorbid Personality

Interpersonal relationships

Use of leisure time

Predominant mood

Attitude to self and others

Attitude to work and responsibility

Religious beliefs and moral attitudes

Fantasy life

Habits

PHYSICAL EXAMINATION

S. No.	Vital sign	Normal value	Patient's value
1.	Temperature	98.6°F	
2.	Pulse	72–90 beats/min	
3.	Respiration	14–20 breath/min	
4.	Blood pressure	120/80 mm Hg	

MENTAL STATUS EXAMINATION

General Appearance and Behavior

Appearance

Level of grooming

Level of cleanliness

Level of consciousness

Mode of entry

Cooperativeness

Eye-to-eye contact

Psychomotor activity

Rapport

Gesturing

Posturing

Other movements

Other catatonic phenomena

Conversion and dissociative signs

Compulsive acts or rituals

Hallucinatory behavior

Inference:

Speech
Student Nurse:

<u>Client</u>
Initiation

Reaction time

Rate

Productivity

___

Volume

___

Tone

___

Relevance

___

Stream

___

Coherence

___

Others

___

Mood

Subjective:

___

Student nurse:

___

Patient:

___

Objective:
Thought

Student Nurse

Client:

Stream

Form

Content

Student nurse:

Client:
Remarks:

Perception

Hallucinations

Student Nurse:

Client:
Remarks:

Cognitive Functions

Consciousness

_____

Student Nurse:

_____

Client:
Remarks

_____

_____

Orientation

_____

Person

_____

Student Nurse:

_____

Client:
Remarks

_____

_____

Student Nurse:

_____

Client:
Remarks

Time

Student Nurse

Client:
Remarks

Attention

Student Nurse:

Client:
Remarks

Practical Record Book of Psychiatric Nursing

Concentration

_____

Student Nurse:

_____

Client:
Remarks

_____

Memory

_____

Immediate

_____

Student Nurse:

_____

Client:
Remarks

_____

Recent

_____

Student Nurse:

_____

Client:
Remarks:

___

___

Remote

___

Student Nurse:

___

Client
Remarks

___

___

Intelligence

___

Student Nurse

___

Client:
Remarks

___

___

Abstraction

___

Student Nurse:

Client:
Remarks

Insight: (grade1 to 6)

Student Nurse:

Client
Remarks

Judgment

Student Nurse:

Client:
Remarks:

INVESTIGATION

Sl. No	Investigations	Patient's value	Normal value
1.	Blood • Heamoglobin • Red blood cell • PCV • Platelets • Total WBC different count • Lymphocytes • Eosinophils • Monocytes • MCV • MCH • MCHC • ESR Routine investigation • RBS • Blood urea • S. creatinine • S. sodium • S. potassium LFT • S. bilirubin • S. total protein • S. albumin • S. globulin • Alkaline phosphate		13–15 4.5–6.51 20–54 1.5–4.5 5000–11000 20–45 1–6 1–6 80–99 27–33 32–37 0–20 <150 20–45 0.7–1.2 135–145 3.5–4.5 1 6–8 3–5 1.8–3.6 80–120

MEDICATION CHART/DRUG SHEET

Sl. No.	Trade name	Pharmacological name	Group	Doses	Route	Frequency	Action	Indication	Contraindications	Side-effects	Nursing responsibility
1.											
2.											
3.											

Contd...

Sl. No.	Trade name	Pharmacological name	Group	Doses	Route	Frequency	Action	Indication	Contraindications	Side-effects	Nursing responsibility
4.											
5.											
6.											

OTHER THERAPEUTIC THERAPIES

Assessment Techniques

Summary

Nursing Process

Nursing Diagnosis

Practical Record Book of Psychiatric Nursing

Nursing diagnose	Goals	Intervention	Implementation	Evaluation

Contd...

Nursing diagnosis	Goals	Planning	Implementation	Evaluation

Contd...

Practical Record Book of Psychiatric Nursing

Nursing diagnosis	Goals	Planning	Implementation	Evaluation

Health Education

Discharge Plan

SUMMARY

BIBLIOGRAPHY

FORMAT OF NURSING CARE PLAN

Format 3

Identification Data

Client name: _____	Age: _____
Sex: _____	Father: _____
Address: _____	Education: _____
Occupation: _____	Income: _____
Marital status: _____	Religion: _____
Date of admission: _____	Diagnosis: _____

Informant

_____
_____
_____
_____

Presenting Chief Complaints

According to Patient

_____
_____
_____
_____

According to Informant

_____
_____
_____
_____

History of Present Illness

_____
_____
_____
_____

Treatment History
___

Past Psychiatric History
___

Past Medical History
___

Past Surgical History
___

Family History
___

Genogram
___

Socio-economic History

Personal History

Prenatal History

Childhood History

Educational History

Play History

Emotional Problems during Adolescence

_____
_____
_____
_____
_____

Puberty

_____
_____
_____
_____

Occupational History

_____
_____
_____
_____
_____
_____

Premorbid Personality

Interpersonal relationships

_____

Use of leisure time

_____

Predominant mood

_____

Attitude to self and others

_____

Attitude to work and responsibility

Religious beliefs and moral attitudes

Fantasy life

Habits

PHYSICAL EXAMINATION

S. No.	Vital sign	Normal value	Patient's value
1.	Temperature	98.6°F	
2.	Pulse	72–90 beats/min	
3.	Respiration	14–20 breath/min	
4.	Blood pressure	120/80 mm Hg	

MENTAL STATUS EXAMINATION

General Appearance and Behavior

Appearance

Level of grooming

Level of cleanliness

Level of consciousness

_____

Mode of entry

_____

Cooperativeness

_____

Eye-to-eye contact

_____

Psychomotor activity

_____

Rapport

_____

Gesturing

_____

Posturing

_____

Other movements

_____

Other catatonic phenomena

_____

Conversion and dissociative signs

Compulsive acts or rituals

Hallucinatory behavior

Inference:

Speech
Student Nurse:

<u>Client</u>
Initiation

Reaction time

Rate

Productivity

_____

Volume

_____

Tone

_____

Relevance

_____

Stream

_____

Coherence

_____

Others

_____

Mood

Subjective:

_____

Student nurse:

_____

Patient:

_____

Objective:
Thought

Student Nurse

Client:

Stream

Form

Content

Student nurse:

Client:
Remarks:

Perception

Hallucinations

Student Nurse:

Client:
Remarks:

Cognitive Functions

Consciousness

_____

Student Nurse:

_____

Client:
Remarks

_____

_____

Orientation

_____

Person

_____

Student Nurse:

_____

Client:
Remarks

_____

_____

Student Nurse:

_____

Client:
Remarks

Time

Student Nurse

Client:
Remarks

Attention

Student Nurse:

Client:
Remarks

Concentration

Student Nurse:

Client:
Remarks

Memory

Immediate

Student Nurse:

Client:
Remarks

Recent

Student Nurse:

Practical Record Book of Psychiatric Nursing

Client:
Remarks:
_____
_____

Remote
_____

Student Nurse:
_____

Client
Remarks
_____
_____

Intelligence
_____

Student Nurse
_____

Client:
Remarks
_____
_____

Abstraction
_____

Student Nurse:

Client:
Remarks

Insight: (grade1 to 6)

Student Nurse:

Client
Remarks

Judgment

Student Nurse:

Client:
Remarks:

INVESTIGATION

Sl. No	Investigations	Patient's value	Normal value
1.	Blood		
	• Heamoglobin		13–15
	• Red blood cell		4.5–6.51
	• PCV		20–54
	• Platelets		1.5–4.5
	• Total WBC different count		5000–11000
	• Lymphocytes		20–45
	• Eosinophils		1–6
	• Monocytes		1–6
	• MCV		80–99
	• MCH		27–33
	• MCHC		32–37
	• ESR		0–20
	Routine investigation		
	• RBS		
	• Blood urea		<150
	• S. creatinine		20–45
	• S. sodium		0.7–1.2
	• S. potassium		135–145
	LFT		3.5–4.5
	• S. bilirubin		
	• S. total protein		1
	• S. albumin		6–8
	• S. globulin		3–5
	• Alkaline phosphate		1.8–3.6
			80–120

MEDICATION CHART/DRUG SHEET

Sl. No.	Trade name	Pharmacological name	Group	Doses	Route	Frequency	Action	Indication	Contraindications	Side-effects	Nursing responsibility
1.											
2.											
3.											

Contd...

Sl. No.	Trade name	Pharmacological name	Group	Doses	Route	Frequency	Action	Indication	Contraindications	Side-effects	Nursing responsibility
4.											
5.											
6.											

OTHER THERAPEUTIC THERAPIES

Assessment Techniques

Summary

Nursing Process

Nursing Diagnosis

Nursing diagnose	Goals	Intervention	Implementation	Evaluation

Contd...

Nursing diagnosis	Goals	Planning	Implementation	Evaluation

Contd...

Nursing diagnosis	Goals	Planning	Implementation	Evaluation

Contd...

Health Education

Discharge Plan

SUMMARY

BIBLIOGRAPHY

EXAMPLE OF CASE STUDY

BIODATA OF THE PATIENT

Name : Inderpal
Sex : Male
Ward : male closed ward
Religion : Hindu
Occupation: Unemployed
D.O.A: 24/10/2018
Informant: Mrs. Shobha and Ms. Sonika
Reliability of informant: Reliable

Age : 30 years
Reg. No. : 2009-10-37232
Marital status: Unmarried
Education: B.A
Language: Hindi
Diagnosis: Paranoid schizophrenia
Relationship with patient : mother and sister

PRESENTING COMPLAINTS

According to the Patient:

- Mujhe kuch acha nhi lgta tha.
- Gussa bahut aata tha.
- Log tarah-2 ki baatein krte the mere bare me.
- Mere peeche police laga di thi, jhuthi complaint kr k jo mujhe maarna chahti thi.

ACCORDING TO RELATIVES:

Patient was presented to the hospital with C/O:
- Suspiciousness
- Withdrawn behavior
- Aggressiveness
- Decreased socialization
- Muttering to self
- Crying spells
- Irregular sleep and appetite.

HISTORY OF PRESENT ILLNESS

Onset of illness is insidious. The patient was apparently well till about 25 years of his age, while in last year of his graduation, his behavior changed. He became irregular at college and started spending more time at home. After his father's death he became more emotionally disturbed. His treatment was started from RML Hospital, Delhi. Whenever he delayed his medicine, his behavior became bizarre. He used to suspect his mother and sister and was fully sure that they have launched a false complaint against him in the police station for teasing a girl. He became aggressive but there was peak social withdrawal. He refused food and also his personal hygiene decreased. One day he just tried to stab his neighbor just because of suspiciousness. After that he was bought to IHBAS where he was admitted by his mother's will.

PAST HISTORY OF ILLNESS

MEDICAL: No H/O Diabetes mellitus
No H/O Tuberculosis

No H/O Hypertension
No H/O Jaundice
SURGICAL: Nothing significant

PSYCHIATRIC HISTORY: The patient was apparently well till about 25 years of his age, while in last year of his graduation, his behavior changed. He became irregular at college and started spending more time at home. He remained lost in his own thoughts and became irritable on small issues. Gradually he stopped interacting with friends and family members. He became suspicious and would always suspect his mother and sister that they are making plans for killing him. His condition deteriorated 3 years ago after his father's death. After this he was taken to RML Hospital for treatment. He showed good compliance and improvement with medicine. But according to patient's sister, from last few months, the patient was not taking the prescribed dose of his medicine, irritability increased and also there was increase in his suspicious behavior. So, he was admitted to IHBAS under section 19(1) of mental health act as sister and mother of the patient considered him to be mentally ill and desired him to be admitted in the hospital.

FAMILY HISTORY

Patient lived with his mother and sisters who are settled in Delhi. Patient has two sisters and one of which is married. Patient is unmarried. There is no significant family history of medical, surgical or psychiatric illness

PERSONAL HISTORY

Birth And Early Development: Patient was born by full term normal vaginal delivery in hospital with no pre natal; natal and post natal complications. Patient gasped and cried soon after birth. He had normal milestones and development.
Childhood: No H/O any behavioral disorder. Started schooling at the age of 3 years. Patient was an intelligent student in his school life.
Physical Illness During Childhood: There is no significant history of physical illness during childhood.
School: Patient started her schooling at 3 years of age. His performance in school was good and patient had interest in studies. Patient had good relationship with her peers as well as teachers.
Occupation: Patient was unemployed.
Sexual History: Normal onset of puberty.
Marital History: Patient is unmarried.
Substance Abuse: No H/O substance abuse

PRE MORBID PERSONALITY

Social Relations: Patient had developed suspicious nature towards her family members and relatives.
Intellectual Activities: Patient's hobbies include reading novels, watching T.V.
Mood: Patient had stable mood and used to behave in normal pattern.
Habits: When patient was not having suspicious nature he was having good relation with his family and friends and was fond of playing cricket and playing cards.

MENTAL STATUS EXAMINATION

Appearance

- Grooming and dress: Patient is wearing appropriate dress which is according to the place and season. Patient is wearing shirt, trouser, sweater and shoes.
- Hygiene : Hygienic condition of the patient is good. Clothes of patient are clean. Nails of the patient are clean and are cut properly. Hairs are combed.
- Physique: Patient is of average built and height.

- Posture: Patient is having an open posture. He is sitting upright on a chair.
- Facial expressions:
  - Patient is attentive.
  - Facial expressions are appropriate and consistent with the subject under discussion.
  - Patient shows mild pleasure at times.
- Level of eye contact: Patient maintains eye-to-eye contact almost throughout the conversation.
- Rapport: A comfortable rapport is maintained with the patient. He took part in the conversation well and responded to all the questions asked to him.

Motor Activity:

- Patient's level of activity is normal.

Speech:

- Patient speaks in Hindi and English. Rate of speech is normal and he speaks in normal volume. Content of speech is appropriate.

Emotions

- Mood: Patient feels better. He is in a normal mood.
- Affect: Patient's emotional response is congruent with the speech content.

Thought

- Formation level: Formation level of the patient is intact.
- Content level: Content level of thought is also impaired, as patient is having delusion of persecution, delusion of grandiosity and delusion of reference.
- Progression level: Progression level of thought is intact.

Perception

N-Kya aapko koi awaze sunai deti hai Jo aapke saath baatain kar rahi ho
P: Haan pehle hoti thi abhi nahi.
N: Aapko koi smell to nahi AA rahi hai
P: Nahi

Inference

Perception in patient is intact. Patient is not having any kind of hallucinations or illusions at present. There is history of auditory hallucinations.

Sensorium and Cognitive Ability

- Level of alertness/consciousness: Patient is alert and conscious. He actively listens to all the questions and answers them as per his knowledge and skills.
- Orientation: Patient is fully oriented to place, person and time.
- Memory
  - **Immediate memory:** Immediate memory intact.
  - **Recent memory:** Recent memory intact.
  - **Remote memory:** Patient's remote memory is impaired.
- Concentration and attention: Patient is having good concentration and attention.
- Information and intelligence: Patients' information and intelligence is impaired.

- Abstract thinking : Abstract thinking of the patient is good.
- Judgment
  - **Social:** Patient has logical social judgment.
  - **Persona:** Patient has fair personal judgment.

Insight

- Insight is absent. Patient has grade -I rating score.

General Attitude

- Patient is in normal mood. He is communicating well. He is very co-operative.

Special Points

N: Is your appetite good?
P: yes
N: Do you sleep appropriately?
P: Yes.
N: Do you have any bowel problems?
P: No.
Inference: Patient's appetite and sleep patterns are normal

DIAGNOSIS: PARANOID SCHIZOPHRENIA

What is paranoid schizophrenia: Paranoid schizophrenia is characterized by predominantly positive symptoms of schizophrenia, including delusions and hallucinations. These debilitating symptoms blur the line between what is real and what isn't, making it difficult for the person to lead a typical life.

Causes:

In book	In patient
It's not known what causes schizophrenia, but researchers believe that a combination of genetics, brain chemistry and environment contributes to development of the disorder.	Cause is not known in his case.

Symptoms:

In book	In patient
Delusions of persecution, reference, grandeur, control, or infidelity. The delusions are usually well systematized (i.e. thematically well connected with each other).	Delusion of persecution and reference
The hallucinations usually have a persecutory or grandiose content.	Persecutory hallucinations
Disturbances of affect volition speech and motor behavior.	Absent

The onset of paranoid schizophrenia is usually insidious occurs later in life as compared to the other types of schizophrenias. The course is usually progressive and complete recovery usually does not occur.

MANAGEMENT OF SCHIZOPHRENIA/ TREATMENT METHODS OF SCHIZOPHRENIA

Medical Management

Somatic (Physical) Therapies

- ☐ Yoga Therapy
- ☐ Group Therapy
- ☐ Carrom Playing
- ☐ Exercise

Antipsychotic Medications

Drug	Oral dose (mg/day)	For patient
TYPICAL OR TRADITIONAL ANTIPSYCHOTICS		
• Chlorpromazine	300-1500	
• Thioridazine	300-800	✓
• Trifluoperazine	15-60	
• Haloperidol	5-100	
• Pimozide	4-12	
• Triflupromazine	100-400	
• Prochlorperazine	45-150	
• Flupenthixol	3-10	
• Lolapine	25-150	
• Zudopenthixol	50-150	
ATYPICAL OR NEWER ANTIPSY CHOTICS		
• Clozapine	25-450	✓
• Resperidone	2-8	
• Olanzapine	5-20	✓
• Ziprasidone	40-160	

ECT (Electro – Convulsive Therapy)

In book	In patient
Schizophrenia is not a primary indication for ECT. Indications for ECT in schizophrenia include: • Catatonic stupor • Uncontrolled catatonic excitement • A cute exacerbation not controlled with drugs. • Severe side effect with drugs in presence of untreated schizophrenia	Not prescribed in his case till date.

Psychological Treatment

In book	In patient
• Hospitalization	✓
• Psychotherapy	Not prescribed in his case till date.
• Rehabilitation - social, vocational	✓
• Aftercare – day treatment, halfway homes	Not prescribed in his case till date
• Education about illness for patients and families	✓

NURSING MANAGEMENT OF PARANOID SCHIZOPHRENIA

Disrupted Sensory Perception (Auditory/Visual)

Usually evidenced by:

☐ Altered speech pattern
☐ Inability to concentrate
☐ Disoriented
☐ Incongruent responses
☐ Hallucinations
☐ Talking, murmuring or laughing to self
☐ Frequent blinking of the eyes and frowning
☐ Observable change in sensory alertness

Nursing Interventions	Rationale
Acknowledge that the voices and sightings are real to the client but clearly state that you do not hear or see them.	Stating to the client that you do not sense or perceive the voices and sightings will help the client become uncertain of the validity of what he/she sees or hears.
Look into how the hallucinations are experienced by the client.	Exploring the hallucinations with the client will help him/her gain a sense of being empowered, thus improving the chances of the client being able to manage his/her hallucinations.
Whenever possible, decrease environmental stimuli.	This will decrease potential for anxiety which can trigger hallucinations. Decreased stimuli will help the client calm down.
Make conversations simple, basic and reality-based. Avoid bombarding client with multiple ideas. Instead help the client to focus on one idea at a time.	The client's thought process might be disorganized. A basic and reality-based conversation will help the client to focus.
Involve the client in reality-based activities such as drawing or listening to music.	Being engaged in reality-based activity provides a healthy diversion and prevents the client from acting out his/her hallucinations.
Stay with the client when he/she starts to hallucinate. Guide him/her to tell the "voices" to go away. Repeat this often and in a tone that is matter-of-fact.	There are instances when clients can learn to push away or disregard the voices when they are given repeated instructions.
If voices predispose a client to self-harm or harming others, take the necessary environmental precautions. Be sure to follow the given protocol on this.	Clients usually obey hallucinatory commands even those involving killing self or others. Proper intervention will help save lives.
Intervene with medication (as needed) or one on one seclusion when appropriate. Be sure to follow protocol.	This will prevent the client's level of anxiety from escalating, thereby keeping the patient from being out of control.
Guide the client in identifying activities that help reduce his/her anxiety.	This will help the client lessen his/her anxiety, while also helping the nurse to build rapport with the client.

Impaired Social Interaction

Usually evidenced by:
- ☐ Inability to make eye contact
- ☐ Inability to begin or respond to social conversations
- ☐ Inappropriate emotional response
- ☐ Prefers to be alone
- ☐ Exhibits behavior or verbalizes discomfort in social situations
- ☐ Noted use of ineffective social interactions

Nursing Interventions	Rationale
Identify with client symptoms he/she experiences when he/she begins to feel anxious around others.	Identification of the symptoms of anxiety will help decrease agitation and aggression of the client.
Avoid touching the client.	This is particularly applies to a paranoid client. Touch especially by an unknown person can be misinterpreted as sexual or viewed as threatening by the client.
Minimize stimuli (avoid loud noises or crowding) as much as possible.	Noise and a huge crowd might result to the client feeling agitated and anxious.
Structure activities based on the client's pace and abilities.	The client might be disinterested in activities that he/she finds overwhelming. This will ten lead to an increased sense of failure.
Structure times that include planned brief interactions and activities with the client on a one-on-one basis.	This will help the client develop a sense of safety in a non-threatening environment.
Check if the medications have reached therapeutic levels.	Many symptoms of schizophrenia subside with medications. This in turn helps facilitate interactions.
If the client is extremely paranoid, solitary or one-on-one activities are appropriate. Said activities must require a degree of concentration.	The client has the freedom to choose his/her level of interaction. However, encouraging him/her to concentrate can help minimize distressing paranoid thoughts or hallucinations.
Encourage the client to use coping skills particularly conversational and assertiveness abilities.	This will help the client develop the fundamental skills in socializing.
Remember to give praise or recognition for positive steps the client takes in increasing social skills.	Recognition and appreciation encourages the client to sustain and increase a specific social behavior.
Involve the client in social skills training.	This type of training help the client to adapt and function in the society thereby increasing his/her quality of life.

Interrupted Family Process

Usually evidenced by:
- ☐ Altered communication patters in the family
- ☐ Changes in stress reduction behavior
- ☐ Lack of mutual support
- ☐ Knowledge deficit on community and healthcare support
- ☐ Knowledge deficit on the disease

Nursing Interventions	Rationale
Assess the family's level of knowledge about the disease.	Family members might have misconceptions about the disease. This might lead to their inability to deal with the situation.
Discuss clearly with the client's family the course of treatment such as psychopharmacologic therapy. Written information should also be given to the client and his/her family.	This will foster family support and improve client adherence to treatment.
Determine the family's coping abilities (e.g. role of a care giver; experience of loss).	This helps stabilize the family unit.
Provide health teachings to the client and his/her family (e.g. signs and symptoms of relapse)	This helps the family to recognize early warning symptoms which is vital in preventing relapse.
Provide an opportunity for the family to discuss feelings related to the ill member of the family. Try to identify their immediate concerns.	Being able to express how they feel will help the family in coping with the situation. This will also enable the nurse to properly help the family in their struggle to cope.
Provide information to client and family regarding community resources and organizations.	Knowing about community resources and organizations will help the client and his/her family to cope with the situation. This will minimize isolation.

SUMMARY

Client is having paranoid schizophrenia characterized by Delusion of persecution and reference and persecutory hallucination. He is socially withdrawn and on antipsychotics.

Practical Record Book of Psychiatric Nursing

FORMAT OF CASE STUDY

Format 1

BIODATA OF THE PATIENT

Name: _____   Age: _____

Sex: _____   Reg. no. _____

Ward: _____   Marital status: _____

Religion: _____   Education: _____

Occupation: _____   Language: _____

D.O.A: _____   Diagnosis: _____

Informant: _____   Relationship with patient: _____

Reliability of informant: _____

PRESENTING COMPLAINTS

According to the Patient:

_____

_____

_____

_____

_____

_____

_____

ACCORDING TO RELATIVES:

_____

_____

_____

_____

_____

HISTORY OF PRESENT ILLNESS

_____

PAST HISTORY OF ILLNESS
Medical:

_____

Surgical:

_____

PSYCHIATRIC HISTORY:

_____

FAMILY HISTORY

_____
_____

PERSONAL HISTORY

Birth And Early Development:

_____
_____

Childhood:

_____
_____

Physical Illness During Childhood:

_____
_____

School:

_____
_____

Occupation:

_____
_____

Sexual History:

_____
_____

Marital History:

_____

Substance Abuse:

_____
_____

PRE MORBID PERSONALITY

Social Relations:

_____
_____
_____

Intellectual Activities:

_____
_____
_____

Mood:

_____
_____
_____

Habits:

_____
_____
_____

MENTAL STATUS EXAMINATION

APPEARANCE

1. Grooming and dress:
_____

2. Hygiene :
_____

3. Physique
_____

4. Posture:
_____

5. Facial expressions:
_____

6. Level of eye contact:
_____

7. Rapport:
_____

MOTOR ACTIVITY:

SPEECH:
___
___

EMOTIONS

1. Mood
___
___

AFFECT:

THOUGHT

1. Formation level:
___

2. Content level:
___

3. Progression level:
___

PERCEPTION

Question 1
___
Answer
___

Question 2
___
Answer
___

Question 3
___
Answer
___

Inference

SENSORIUM AND COGNITIVE ABILITY

Level of Alertness/Consciousness:

Orientation :

Memory

- Immediate memory:

- Recent memory:

- Remote memory:

Concentration and attention:

Information and intelligence:

Abstract thinking :

Judgment

- Social :

- Personal:

INSIGHT

GENERAL ATTITUDE

SPECIAL POINTS

N:

P:

N:

P:

N:

P:

Inference:

DIAGNOSIS:

MANAGEMENT/TREATMENT METHODS

Medical Management

Somatic (Physical) Therapies

_____
_____
_____
_____
_____

Antipsychotic Medications

Drugs as per book	Oral dose (mg/day)	For patient

ECT (Electro – Convulsive Therapy)

In book	In patient

Psychological Treatment

In book	In patient

NURSING MANAGEMENT

SUMMARY:

FORMAT OF CASE STUDY

Format 2

BIODATA OF THE PATIENT

Name: _____ Age: _____

Sex: _____ Reg. no. _____

Ward: _____ Marital status: _____

Religion: _____ Education: _____

Occupation: _____ Language: _____

D.O.A: _____ Diagnosis: _____

Informant: _____ Relationship with patient: _____

Reliability of informant: _____

PRESENTING COMPLAINTS

According to the Patient:

_____
_____
_____
_____
_____
_____
_____
_____

ACCORDING TO RELATIVES:

_____
_____
_____
_____
_____

HISTORY OF PRESENT ILLNESS

PAST HISTORY OF ILLNESS

Medical:

Surgical:

PSYCHIATRIC HISTORY:

FAMILY HISTORY

PERSONAL HISTORY

Birth And Early Development:

Childhood:

Physical Illness During Childhood:

School:

Occupation:

Sexual History:

Marital History:

Substance Abuse:

PRE MORBID PERSONALITY

Social Relations:

_____
_____
_____

Intellectual Activities:

_____
_____
_____

Mood:

_____
_____

Habits:

_____
_____

MENTAL STATUS EXAMINATION

APPEARANCE

1. Grooming and dress:
   _____
2. Hygiene :
   _____
3. Physique
   _____
4. Posture:
   _____
5. Facial expressions:
   _____
6. Level of eye contact:
   _____
7. Rapport:
   _____

MOTOR ACTIVITY:

SPEECH:

EMOTIONS

1. Mood

AFFECT:

THOUGHT

1. Formation level:

---

2. Content level:

---

3. Progression level:

PERCEPTION

Question 1

Answer

Question 2

Answer

Question 3

Answer

Inference

SENSORIUM AND COGNITIVE ABILITY

Level of Alertness/Consciousness:

Orientation :

Memory

- Immediate memory:

- Recent memory:

- Remote memory:

Concentration and attention:

Information and intelligence:

Abstract thinking :

Judgment

- Social :

- Personal:

INSIGHT

GENERAL ATTITUDE

SPECIAL POINTS

N:

P:

N:

P:

N:

P:

Inference:

DIAGNOSIS:

MANAGEMENT/TREATMENT METHODS

Medical Management

Somatic (Physical) Therapies

_____
_____
_____
_____
_____

Antipsychotic Medications

Drugs as per book	Oral dose (mg/day)	For patient

ECT (Electro – Convulsive Therapy)

In book	In patient

Psychological Treatment

In book	In patient

NURSING MANAGEMENT

SUMMARY:

EXAMPLE OF CASE PRESENTATION

Follow the instructions to collect information about the client:
- Make rapport with the client.
- Use listening and observation while communicating with the client.
- Spend 45 min. to 1 hour with the patient.
- Try to collect information directly from client and where any doubt about any statement, confirm from family members.
- Use therapeutic communication techniques.
- Read the case file of patient.
- Get information from the staff on duty.
- Get information from the patients of his ward.
- Do not write while communicating with client.

SAMPLE CASE PRESENTATION

Demographic Details

Mr. Kishor is a 27 year old male referred to the Deaddiction Centre following a positive test for Opium at his work place. He works in the Police Department. He currently lives alone in his apartment as his wife left him 3 years back. He has no children from his marriage. He denies any particular religious or spiritual orientation. He speaks Hindi, Punjabi and English, and he reports associating primarily with people who speak Hindi.

Key Findings

The client denies using opium. He says he was at a party where some people were smoking and in hailing, and that he must have tested positive because of their use. He acknowledges drinking several beers at parties like these, but denies that alcohol is an issue for him. He says he does not know why his wife left him other than that he is abusing her. His longest employment is about four years—on his present job. He says he is willing to complete a drug Deaddiction program but insists that he does not have any problems that need attention.

Background

The client was raised primarily by his mother and older sisters after his father left the family when the client was about four. He did not see his father much after that. He reports average grades in school. He did not finish college and has not completed graduation. He has had several jobs, all of which apparently involved manual labor before joining police department. He has never been in treatment.

Formulation

The client's ways of thinking are consistent with his culture. Whether or not he actually uses opium, he denies a problem. He may have issues with intimacy related to his father's abandonment and as evidenced by his relationship with his wife. The pattern of employment and the relationships with his wife suggest poor interpersonal skills.

Interventions and Plan

I attempted to develop rapport through the use of active listening and reflection. The plan is to continue assessment, and through motivational interviewing, attempt to identify an area that the client considers a concern. Allow him to participate in an outpatient group therapy session to avoid adverse consequences at work, to enhance the likelihood that he will learn some new social skills, and to give opportunity to form a new social network.

Reasons for Presentation

Although this case appears routine, I am concerned that I may be overlooking something or that a different formulation of the case might produce a better chance for a positive outcome.

Practical Record Book of Psychiatric Nursing

FORMAT OF CASE PRESENTATION

Demographic Details

Key Findings

Background

Formulation

Interventions and Plan

Reasons for Presentation

ACTIVITY PLANNED BY STUDENTS

ACTIVITY PLANNED BY STUDENTS

ACTIVITY PLANNED BY STUDENTS

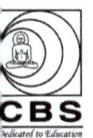
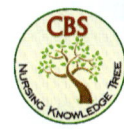

CBS PGMEE & Nursing Division

(A Unit of CBS Publishers & Distributors Pvt. Ltd.)

Nursing Catalogue 2020

Nursing Competitive Exams, Nursing Textbooks, Record Books

Update: November, 2020

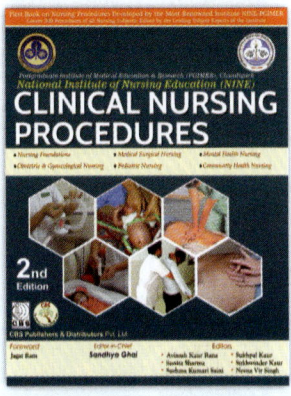

ISBN: 978-93-89261-97-4
Pages: 1296   2/e, 2019

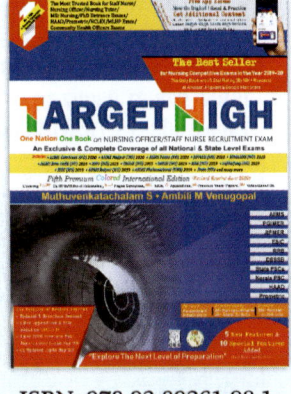

ISBN: 978-93-89261-98-1
Pages: 1350   5/e, 2020-21

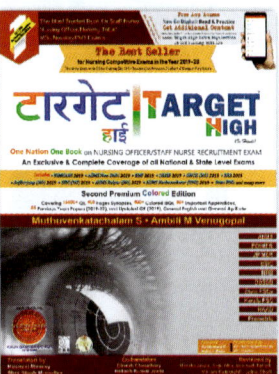

ISBN: 978-81-94025-65-8
Pages: 1296   2/e, 2020

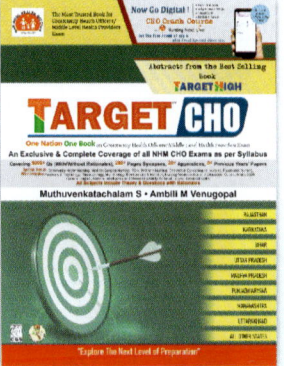

ISBN: 978-81-940256-0-3
Pages: 470   1/e, 2020

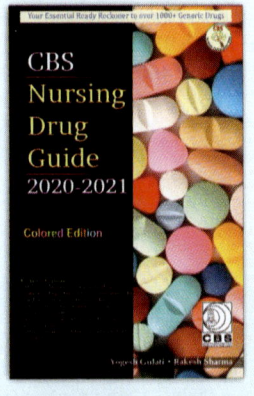

ISBN: 978-93-88178-53-2
Pages: 1670   1/e, 2020

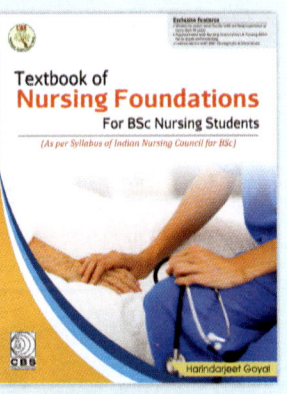

ISBN: 978-93-88108-94-2
Pages: 700   1/e, 2020

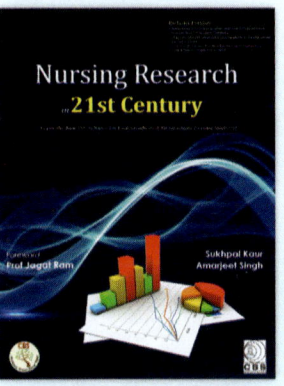

ISBN: 978-93-89261-89-9
Pages: 700   1/e, 2020

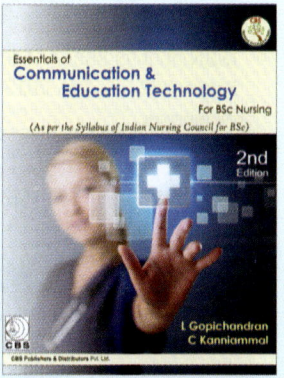

ISBN: 978-93-88178-58-7
Pages: 325   2/e, 2019

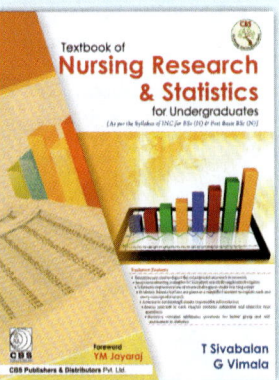

ISBN: 978-93-88178-61-7
Pages: 290   1/e, 2018

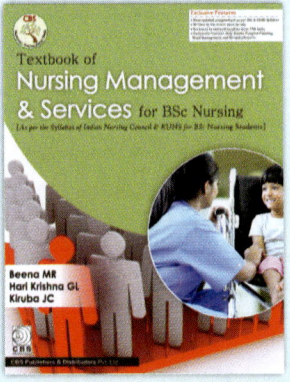

ISBN: 978-93-88178-62-4
Pages: 240   1/e, 2019

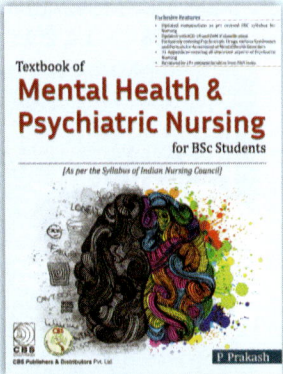

ISBN: 978-93-89261-91-2
Pages: 500   1/e, 2019

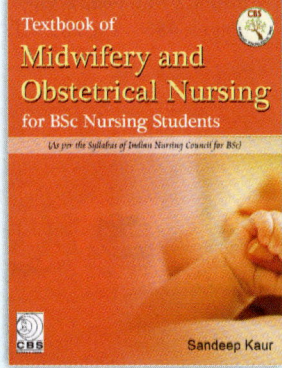

ISBN: 978-93-89261-90-5
Pages: 700 (T)   1/e, 2020

Nursing Competitive Titles/Textbooks for BSc Nursing

Read, Review & Buy

Now, buying CBS Nursing Books is extra convenient with **Nursing Next Live** Mobile App.
Get a Glimpse of **Sample Pages, TOC** before you proceed to buy book.

Download the App from Google Play or scan here to download

Nursing Textbooks for BSc Nursing

CBS PGMEE & Nursing Division

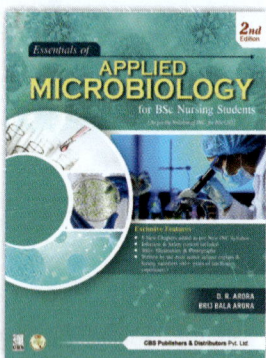

ISBN: 978-81-945234-4-4
Pages: 360 2/e, 2020-21

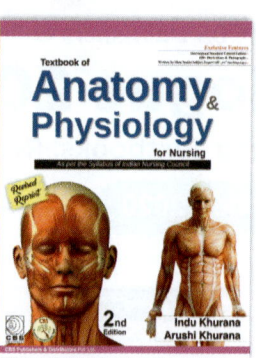

ISBN: 978-93-86827-12-8
Pages: 568 2/e, 2018

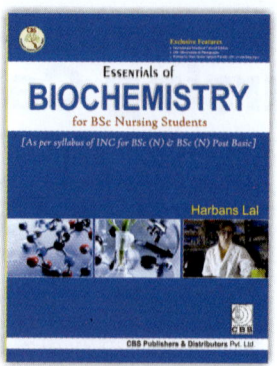

ISBN: 978-81-23927-19-0
Pages: 332 1/e (R/R), 2020-21

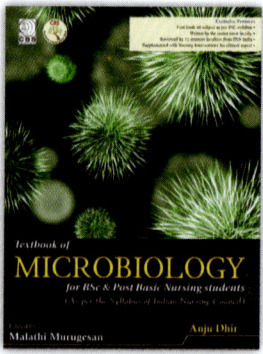

ISBN: 978-93-88108-82-9
Pages: 535 1/e, 2019

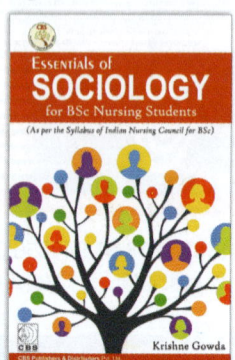

ISBN: 978-93-86217-51-6
Pages: 362 1/e, 2017

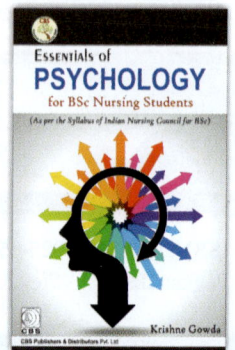

ISBN: 978-81-23927-11-4
Pages: 362 1/e, 2017-18

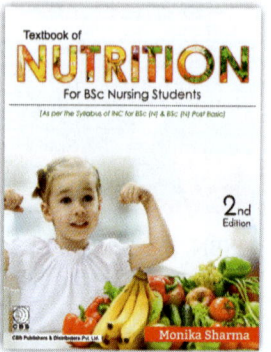

ISBN: 978-93-89261-92-9
Pages: 330 2/e, 2019

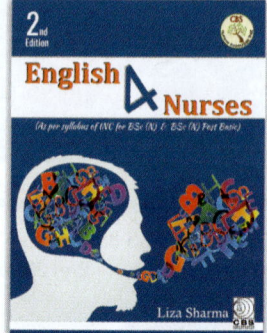

ISBN: 978-93-89261-95-0
Pages: 460 2/e, 2019

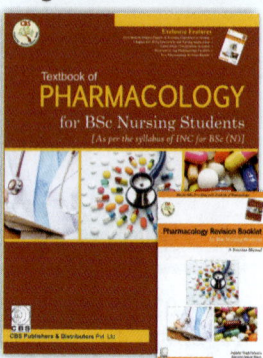

ISBN: 978-93-86217-80-6
Pages: 486 1/e, 2017-18

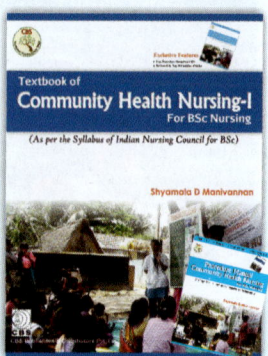

ISBN: 978-81-23927-01-5
Pages: 508 1/e, 2018

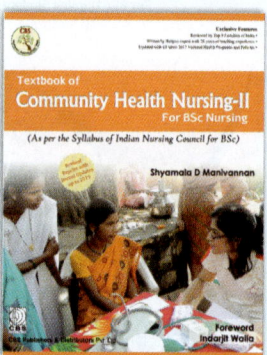

ISBN: 978-93-86827-22-7
Pages: 326 1/e, 2018

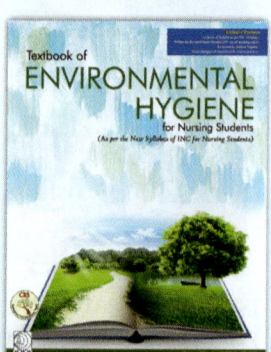

ISBN: 978-93-88178-56-3
Pages: 110 1/e, 2018-19

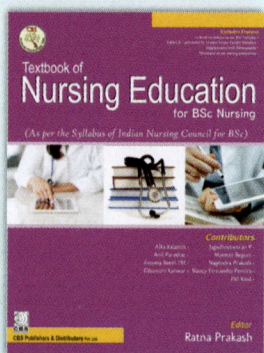

ISBN: 978-93-86827-34-0
Pages: 340 1/e, 2018

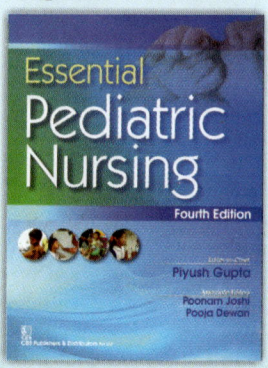

ISBN: 978-93-86217-87-5
Pages: 576 4/e, 2017

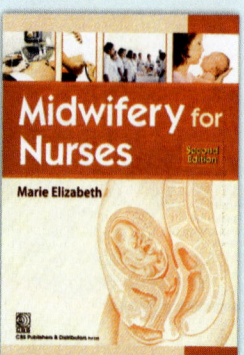

ISBN: 978-81-23922-14-0
Pages: 544 2/e, 2018

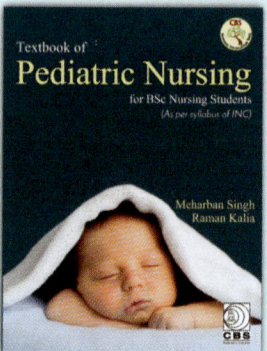

ISBN: 978-93-88108-72-0
Pages: 630 1/e, 2018

Buy online :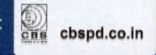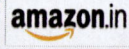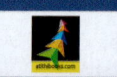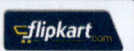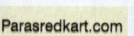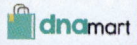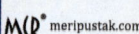

CBS PGMEE & Nursing Division

Nursing Textbooks for BSc Nursing

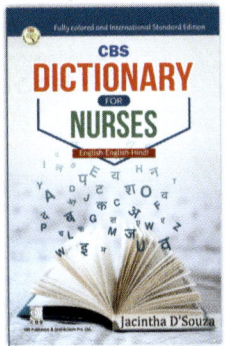
Releasing Soon

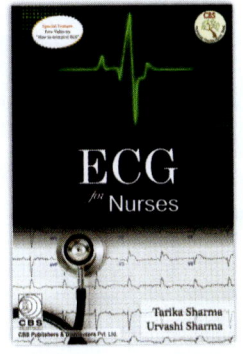
ISBN: 978-93-89261-88-2
Pages: 190   1/e, 2019

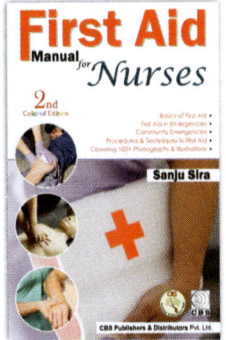
ISBN: 978-93-88178-55-6
Pages: 212   2/e, 2019

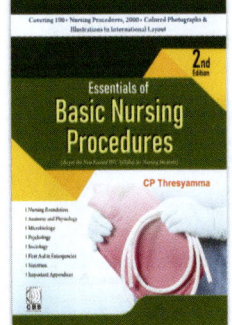
ISBN: 978-81-94523-47-5
Pages: 1016   2/e, 2020

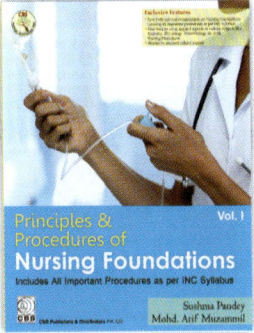
ISBN: 978-93-88108-95-9
Pages: 392   1/e, 2018

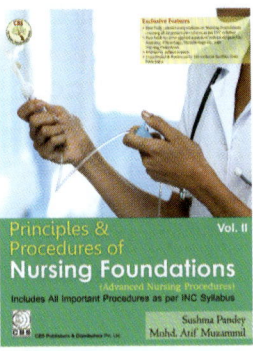
ISBN: 978-93-89261-87-5
Pages: 272   1/e, 2019

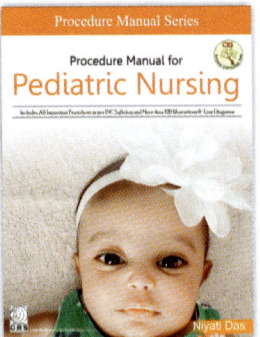
ISBN: 978-93-88108-86-7
Pages: 235   1/e, 2018

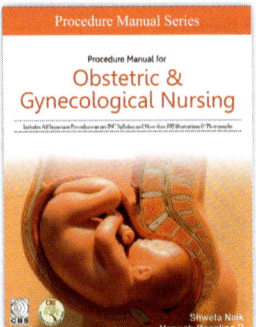
ISBN: 978-93-88178-60-0
Pages: 200   1/e, 2018-19

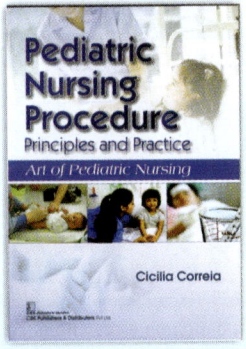
ISBN: 978-93-86310-74-3
Pages: 360   1/e, 2017

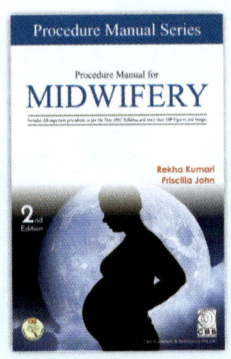
ISBN: 978-93-89261-94-3
Pages: 200   2/e, 2019

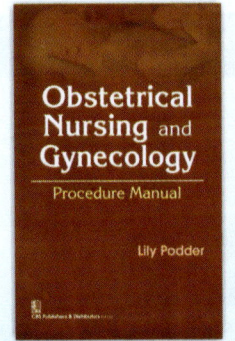
ISBN: 978-81-23925-81-3
Pages: 116   1/e, 2017

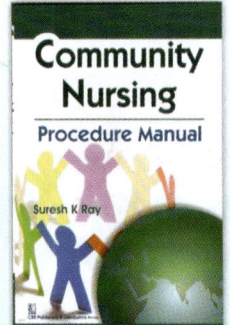
ISBN: 978-81-23929-35-4
Pages: 179   1/e, 2017

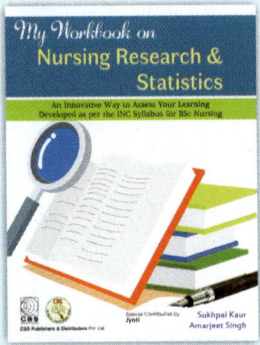
ISBN: 978-93-88108-75-1
Pages: 80   1/e, 2019

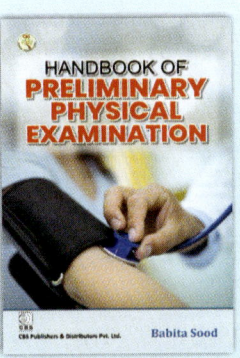
Releasing Soon

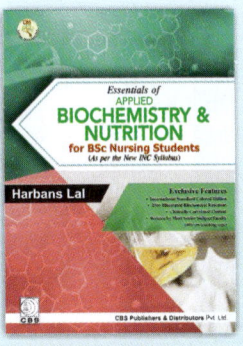
Releasing Soon

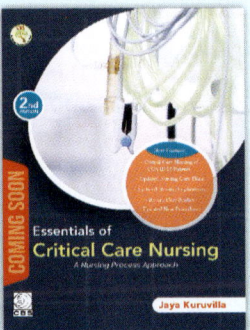
Releasing Soon

Read, Review & Buy
Now, buying CBS Nursing Books is extra convenient with  Mobile App.
Get a Glimpse of **Sample Pages, TOC** before you proceed to buy book.

Offering Best Discount & Offers on all the Books.
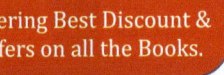

Nursing Textbooks for GNM

CBS PGMEE & Nursing Division

Common Title (BSc/GNM)

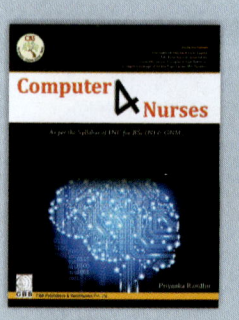
ISBN: 978-93-86310-48-4
Pages: 256   1/e, 2017

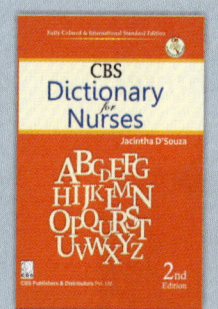
ISBN: 978-81-23927-16-9
Pages: 872   2/e, 2017

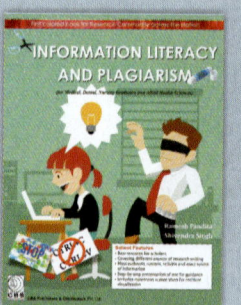
ISBN: 978-93-86827-13-5
Pages: 200   1/e, 2018

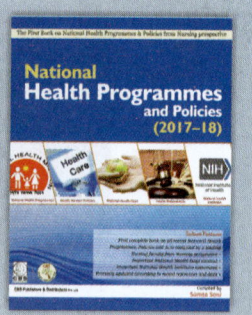
ISBN: 978-93-86310-43-9
Pages: 584   1/e, 2018

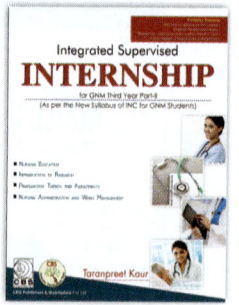
ISBN: 978-93-88108-89-8
Pages: 265   1/e, 2018

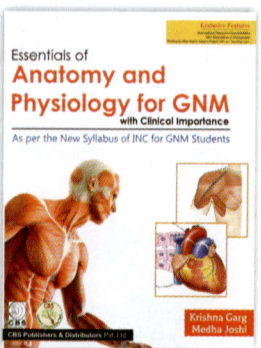
ISBN: 978-93-86827-11-1
Pages: 312   1/e, 2018

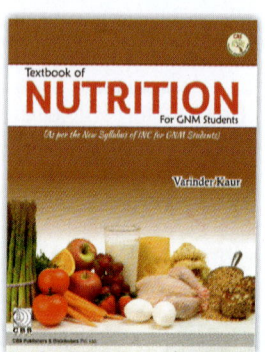
ISBN: 978-93-86827-10-4
Pages: 175   1/e, 2018

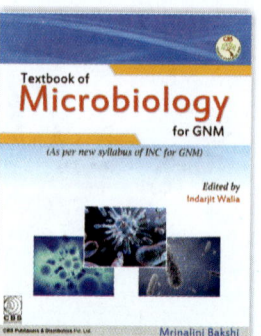
ISBN: 978-93-86827-23-4
Pages: 130   1/e, 2018

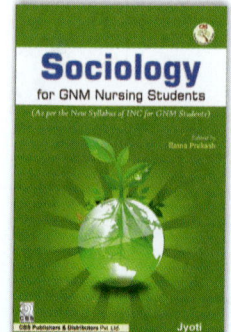
ISBN: 978-93-86827-26-5
Pages: 168   1/e, 2018

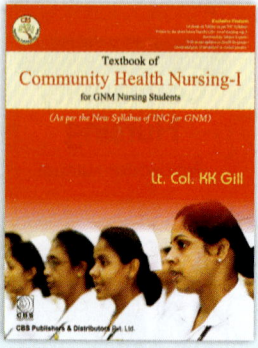
ISBN: 978-93-86827-17-3
Pages: 544   1/e, 2018

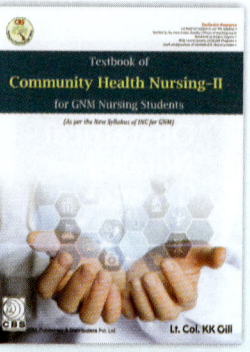
ISBN: 978-93-88178-57-0
Pages: 480   1/e, 2019

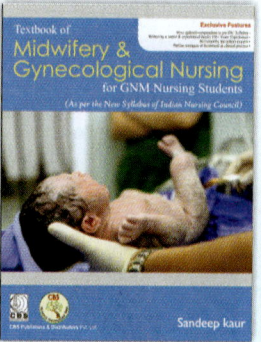
ISBN: 978-93-88108-83-6
Pages: 640   1/e, 2018

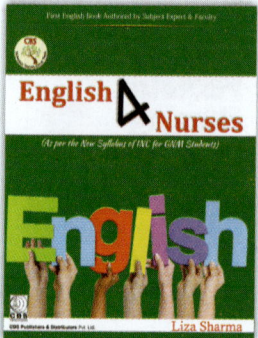
ISBN: 978-93-86827-09-8
Pages: 382   1/e, 2017

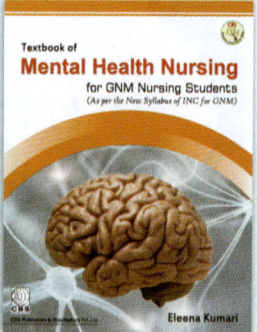
ISBN: 978-93-86827-48-7
Pages: 290   1/e, 2018

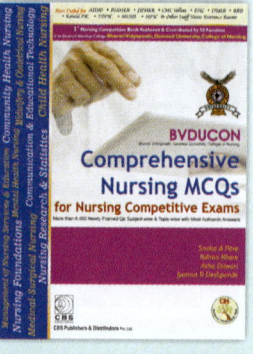
ISBN: 978-93-86310-33-0
Pages: 430   1/e, 2017

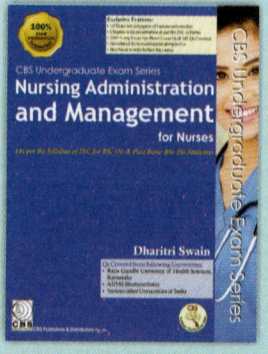
ISBN: 978-93-86827-42-5
Pages: 345   1/e, 2018

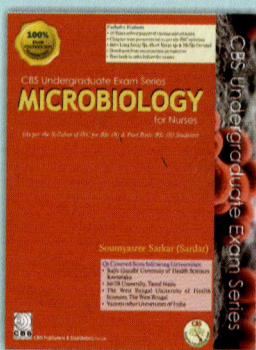
ISBN: 978-93-86310-49-1
Pages: 270   1/e, 2017

Buy online: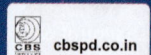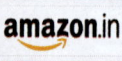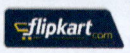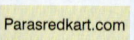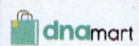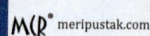

CBS PGMEE & Nursing Division

Nursing Record Books for BSc

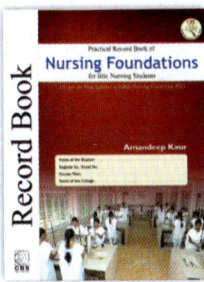
ISBN: 978-93-88108-96-6
Pages: 256   1/e, 2018-19

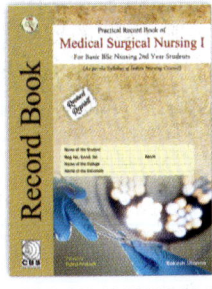
ISBN: 978-81-23928-00-5
Pages: 528   1/e, 2018-19

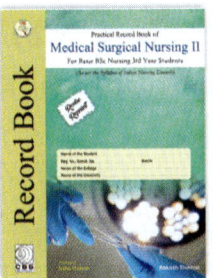
ISBN: 978-81-23928-01-2
Pages: 324   1/e, 2018-19

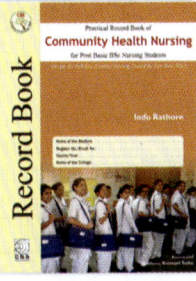
ISBN: 978-93-86827-06-7
Pages: 390   1/e, 2017

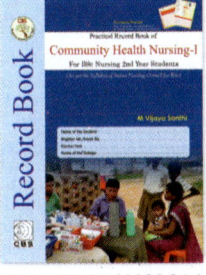
ISBN: 978-81-23926-84-1
Pages: 388   1/e, 2016

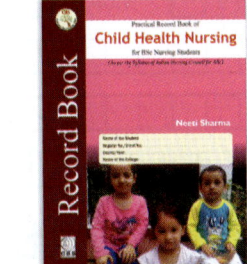
ISBN: 978-93-88108-77-5
Pages: 544   1/e, 2018-19

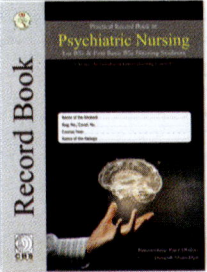
ISBN: 978-93-86827-05-0
Pages: 160   1/e, 2017

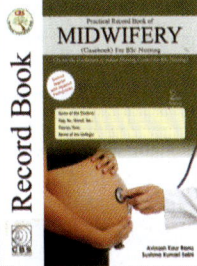
ISBN: 978-93-88108-80-5
Pages: 334   1/e, 2019

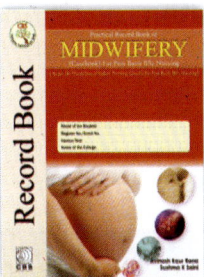
ISBN: 978-93-88178-65-5
Pages: 634   2/e (R/R), 2018-19

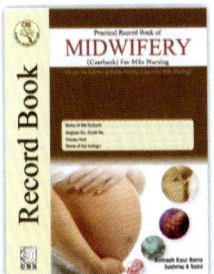
ISBN: 978-81-23927-07-7
Pages: 570   1/e, 2017

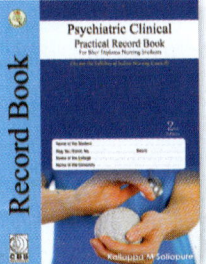
ISBN: 978-93-86217-97-4
Pages: 464   1/e, 2017

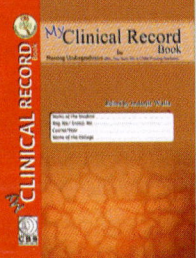
ISBN: 978-93-88108-81-2
Pages: 230   2/e, 2018-19

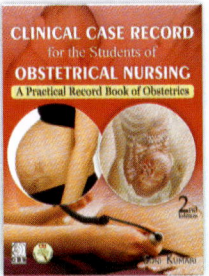
ISBN: 978-81-23927-04-6
Pages: 300   1/e, 2017-18

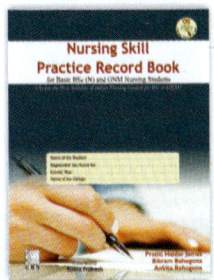
ISBN: 978-93-88178-51-8
Pages: 452   2/e, 2018

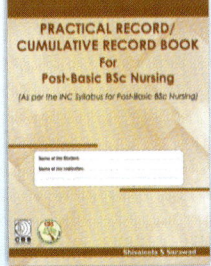
ISBN: 978-93-86827-38-8
Pages: 232   1/e, 2018-19

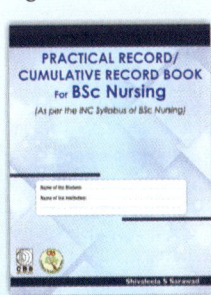
ISBN: 978-93-86827-02-9
Pages: 48   1/e, 2018

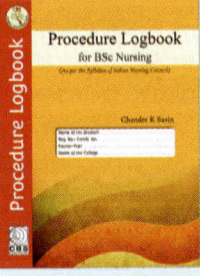
ISBN: 978-93-86827-01-2
Pages: 80   1/e, 2017

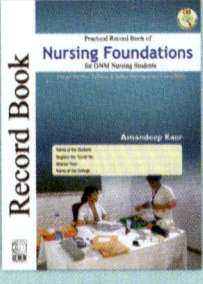
ISBN: 978-93-86310-46-0
Pages: 144   1/e, 2017

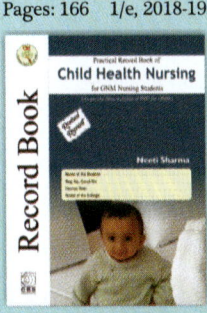
ISBN: 978-93-88178-50-1
Pages: 166   1/e, 2018-19

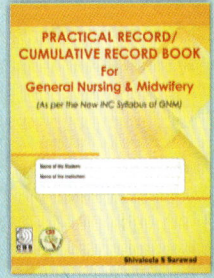
ISBN: 978-93-86827-03-6
Pages: 64   1/e, 2018

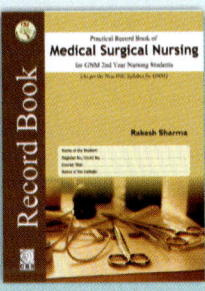
ISBN: 978-93-86827-04-3
Pages: 394   1/e, 2017

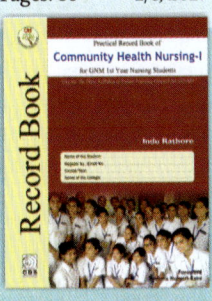
ISBN: 978-93-86827-07-4
Pages: 252   1/e, 2020

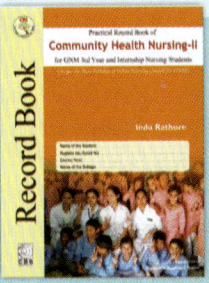
ISBN: 978-93-86827-30-2
Pages: 320   1/e, 2018-19

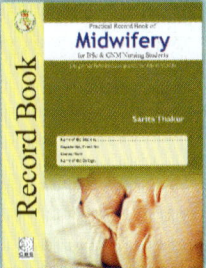
ISBN: 978-93-86827-53-1
Pages: 156   1/e, 2019

ISBN: 978-93-86827-33-3
Pages: 350   1/e, 2020

Read, Review & Buy

Now, buying CBS Nursing Books is extra convenient with Nursing Next Live Mobile App. Get a Glimpse of **Sample Pages, TOC** before you proceed to buy book.

Download the App from Google Play or scan here to download

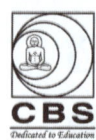
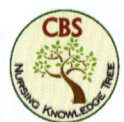

CBS PGMEE & Nursing Division

(A Unit of CBS Publishers & Distributors Pvt. Ltd.)

Sl. No. ☐☐☐☐☐ Date: D D M M Y Y Y Y

College Name: ☐

Contact Person Name: ☐

Email ID: ☐   Mob. No. ☐

Address: ☐

City: ☐ State: ☐ Pin: ☐

Write in Capital Letters

Sl. No.	ISBN	Author	Title	Qty.	Discount
1	9789386827128	Indu Khurana	Textbook of Anatomy & Physiology for Nurses (2/e)		
2	9789388108942	Harindarjeet Goyal	Textbook of Nursing Foundations for BSc Nursing Students		
3	9788123927190	Harbans Lal	Essentials of Biochemistry for BSc Nursing Students		
4	9789389261950	Liza Sharma	English 4 Nurses for BSc(N) and BSc(N) Post Basic (2/e)		
5	9788123927114	Krishne Gowda	Essentials of Psychology for BSc Nursing Students		
6	9788123927138	Arora and Arora	Essentials of Microbiology for BSc Nursing Students		
7	9789388108829	Anju Dhir	Textbook of Microbiology for BSc & Post Basic Nursing Students		
8	9789389261929	Monika Sharma	Textbook of Nutrition for BSc Nursing Students (2/e)		
9	9789388108959	Sushma Pandey/ Mohd. Atif Muzammil	Principles & Procedures of Nursing Foundations (Volume I)		
10	9789389261875	Sushma Pandey/ Mohd. Atif Muzammil	Principles & Procedures of Nursing Foundations (Advanced Nursing Procedures) (Volume II)		
11	9789386310484	Priyanka Randhir	Computer 4 Nurses		
12	9788194523475	CP Thresyamma	Essentials of Basic Nursing Procedures (2/e)		
13	9789389261974	Sandhya Ghai	PGI Nine—Clinical Nursing Procedure (2/e), 2019		
14	9788123927169	Jacintha D'Souza	CBS Dictionary for Nurses		
15	9788123927046	Inderjit Walia	My Clinical Record Book for Nursing Undergraduates		
16	9789388178556	Sanju Sira	First Aid Manual for Nurses (2/e)		
17	9789389261882	Tarika Sharma/ Urvashi Sharma	ECG for Nurses		
18	9789386310460	Chander K Sarin	Procedure Logbook for BSc Nursing		
19	9789386827012	Shivaleela S Sarawad	Practical Record/Cumulative Record Book for BSc Nursing		
20	9789388108966	Amandeep Kaur	Practical Record Book of Nursing Foundation for BSc Nursing Students		
21	9789386217516	Krishne Gowda	Essentials of Sociology for BSc Nursing Students		
22	9789386217806	Joginder Pathania	Textbook of Pharmacology for BSc Nursing Students		
23	9788123927015	Shyamla D Manivannan	Textbook of Community Health Nursing-I		
24	9789388178587	L Gopichandran	Essentials of Communication & Education Technology for BSc Nursing (2/e)		
25	9788123928005	Rakesh Sharma	Medical Surgical Nursing Record Book—2nd Year		
26	9788123926841	M Vijaya Santhi	Practical Record Book of Community Health Nursing-I for BSc Nursing 2nd Year Students		
27	9789386827340	Ratna Prakash	Textbook of Nursing Education for BSc Nursing		
28	9789388178532	Yogesh Gulati, Rakesh Sharma	CBS Nursing Drug Guide 2020-21		
29	9789389261912	P Prakash	Textbook of Mental Health Nursing & Psychiatric Nursing for BSc Students		

Contd...

Sl. No.	ISBN	Author	Title	Qty.	Discount
30	9789388108812	Kallappa M Sollapure	Psychiatric Clinical Practical Record Book for BSc/Diploma Nursing Students		
31	9789386827050	Neeti Sharma	Practical Record Book of Child Health Nursing for BSc Nursing		
32	9788123928012	Rakesh Sharma	Medical Surgical Nursing Record Book-II-3rd Year		
33	9789388108805	Ramandeep Kaur Dhillon	Practical Record Book of Psychiatric Nursing for BSc and PBSc		
34	9789388178655	Avinash Rana	Practical Record Book of Midwifery (Casebook) for BSc Nursing (2/e)		
35	9789388108720	Meharban Singh/ Raman Kalia	Textbook of Pediatric Nursing for BSc Nursing Students		
36	9789388108867	Niyati Das	Procedure Manual for Pediatric Nursing		
37	9789388178518	Soni Kumari	Clinical Case Record for the Students of Obstetrical Nursing (A Practical Record Book of Obstetrics)—(2/e)		
38	9789389261943	Rekha Kumari	Procedure Manual for Midwifery		
39	9789389261899	Sukhpal Kaur, Amarjeet Singh	Nursing Research in 21st Century		
40	9789388108751	Sukhpal Kaur/ Amarjeet Singh	My Workbook on Nursing Research & Statistics		
41	9789388178617	T Sivabalan/G Vimala	Textbook of Nursing Research & Statistics for Undergraduates		
42	9789386217820	Reena J Wani	Textbook of Midwifery for Nurses		
43	9789386827227	Shyamla D Manivannan	Textbook of Community Health Nursing – II for BSc Nursing		
44	9789388178624	Beena MR/ Hari Krishna	Textbook of Nursing Management & Services for BSc Nursing		
45	9789388108775	M Vijaya Santhi	Practical Record Book of Community Health Nursing - II for BSc Nursing 4th Year Students		
46	9788123927077	Avinash Rana	Practical Record Book of Midwifery (for Post Basic BSc Nursing)		
47	9789386310439	Samta Soni	National Health Programmes and Policies (2017-18)		
48	9789388178600	Shweta Naik/ Hannah Roseline D	Procedure Manual for Obstetrics & Gynecological Nursing		
49	9789386827135	Ramesh Pandita/ Shivendra Singh	Information Literacy and Plagiarism		
50	9789386827029	Shivaleela S Sarawad	Practical Record/Cumulative Record Book for Post Basic BSc Nursing		
51	9789386217974	Avinash Kaur Rana/ Sushma Kumari Saini	Practical Record Book of Midwifery (Casebook) for MSc Nursing		
52	9789386827067	Indu Rathor	Practical Record Book of Community Health Nursing for Post BSc Nursing Students		
53	9789386310330	BVDUCON/Sneha A Pitre	BVDUCON Comprehensive Nursing MCQs		
54	9789386310446	Umesh Parashar	Smart Study Nursing Competition Manual		
55	9789386827388	Pratiti Haldar James	Nursing Skill Practical Record Book for Basic BSc(N) & GNM Nursing Students		
56	9789386310491	Soumyashree Sarkar	CBS Undergraduate Exam Series—Microbiology for Nurses		
57	9789386827425	Dharitri Swain	CBS Undergraduate Nursing Administration and Management for Nurses		
58	9789386827111	Krishna Garg/ Medha Josh	Essentials of Anatomy and Physiology for GNM		
59	9789386827104	Varinder Kaur	Textbook of Nutrition for GNM Students		
60	9789386827234	Mrinalini Bakshi	Textbook of Microbiology for GNM		
61	9789386827265	Jyoti	Sociology for GNM Nursing Students		
62	9789388178501	Amandeep Kaur	Practical Record Book of Nursing Foundation for GNM Nursing Students		
63	9789386827098	Liza Sharma	English 4 Nurses for GNM Students		
64	9789386827173	Lt Col. KK Gill	TB of Community Health Nursing-I for GNM		
65	9789386827036	Shivaleela S Sarawad	Practical Record/Cumulative Record Book for GNM Students		
66	9789386827074	Indu Rathor	Practical Record Book of Community Health Nursing-I for GNM 1st Year Nursing Students		
67	9789386827487	Eleena Kumari	Textbook of Mental Health Nursing for GNM Nursing Students		
68	9789388178563	Lt. Col KK Gill	Textbook of Environmental Hygiene for Nursing Students		
69	9789386827043	Rakesh Sharma	Practical Record Book of Medical Surgical Nursing for GNM 2nd Year Students		
70	9789386827302	Indu Rathor	Practical Record Book of Community Health Nurisng - II for GNM 3rd Year & Internship Nursing Students		

Contd...

Sl. No.	ISBN	Author	Title	Qty.	Discount
71	9789388178570	KK Gill	Textbook of Community Health Nursing-II		
72	9789388108836	Sandeep Kaur	Textbook of Midwifery & Gynecological Nursing GNM		
73	9789388108898	Taranpreet Kaur	Integrated Supervised Internship (for GNM-3rd Year)-Part-I		
74	9789386827333	Sarita Thakur	Practical Record Book of Midwifery for GNM Nursing Students		
75	9789386827531	Neeti Sharma	Practical Record Book of Child Health Nursing for GNM Nursing Students		
76	9789389261981	Muthuvenkatachalam	Target High-5th Premium Colored International Edition (5/e)		
77	9788194025658	Muthuvenkatachalam	Target High Hindi (2/e)		
78	9788194025603	Muthuvenkatachalam	Target CHO		
79	9788123929354	Suresh Ray	Community Nursing Procedure Manual		
80	9789386217875	Piyush Gupta	Essential Pediatric Nursing		
81	9789386310743	Cicilia Correia	Pediatric Nursing Procedure Principles and Practice Art of Pediatric Nursing		
82	9788123922140	Marie Elizabeth	Midwifery for Nurses		
83	9788123925813	Lily Poddar	Obstetrical Nursing & Gynaecology		
84	9788194523444	D R Arora, Brij Bala Arora	Essentials of Applied Microbiology for BSc Nursing (2/e), 2020-21		
85	TBA	Jacintha D'Souza	CBS Dictionary for Nurses English-Hinglish-Hindi (1/e), 2020-21		
86	TBA	Babita Sood	Handbook of Preliminary Physical Examination (1/e), 2020-21		
87	TBA	Harbans Lal	Essentials of Applied Biochemistry & Nutrition for BSc Nursing Student (1/e) 2020-21		
88	TBA	Jaya Kuruvilla	Essentials of Critical Care Nursing (2/e), 2020-21		